Complex Trauma Management of the Upper Extremity

Editor

ASIF M. ILYAS

HAND CLINICS

www.hand.theclinics.com

Consulting Editor
KEVIN C. CHUNG

February 2018 • Volume 34 • Number 1

ELSEVIER

1600 John F. Kennedy Boulevard • Suite 1800 • Philadelphia, Pennsylvania, 19103-2899

http://www.theclinics.com

HAND CLINICS Volume 34, Number 1
February 2018 ISSN 0749-0712, ISBN-13: 978-0-323-56982-8

Editor: Lauren Boyle
Developmental Editor: Kristen Helm

Hand Clinics (ISSN 0749-0712) is published quarterly by Elsevier Inc., 360 Park Avenue South, New York, NY 10010-1710. Months of publication are February, May, August, and November. Business and Editorial Offices: 1600 John F. Kennedy Blvd., Ste. 1800, Philadelphia, PA 19103-2899. Customer Service Office: 3251 Riverport Lane, Maryland Heights, MO 63043. Periodicals postage paid at New York, NY and at additional mailing offices. Subscription price is $422.00 per year (domestic individuals), $772.00 per year (domestic institutions), $100.00 per year (domestic students/residents), $481.00 per year (Canadian individuals), $898.00 per year (Canadian institutions), $541.00 per year (international individuals), $898.00 per year (international institutions), and $256.00 per year (international and Canadian students/residents). Foreign air speed delivery is included in all *Clinics* subscription prices. All prices are subject to change without notice. **POSTMASTER:** Send address changes to *Hand Clinics*, Elsevier Health Sciences Division, Subscription Customer Service, 3251 Riverport Lane, Maryland Heights, MO 63043. Customer Service (orders, claims, online, change of address): Elsevier Health Sciences Division, Subscription **Customer Service, 3251 Riverport Lane, Maryland Heights, MO 63043. Tel: 1-800-654-2452 (U.S. and Canada); 314-447-8871 (outside U.S. and Canada). Fax: 314-447-8029. E-mail: journalscustomerservice-usa@elsevier.com (for print support); journalsonlinesupport-usa@elsevier.com (for online support).**

Reprints. For copies of 100 or more of articles in this publication, please contact the Commercial Reprints Department, Elsevier Inc., 360 Park Avenue South, New York, New York 10010-1710. Tel.: 212-633-3874; Fax: 212-633-3820; E-mail: reprints@elsevier.com.

Hand Clinics is covered in *MEDLINE/PubMed (Index Medicus), Current Contents/Clinical Medicine, EMBASE/Excerpta Medica,* and *ISI/BIOMED.*

Contributors

CONSULTING EDITOR

KEVIN C. CHUNG, MD, MS
Chief of Hand Surgery, University of Michigan
Health System, Charles B.G. De Nancrede
Professor of Plastic Surgery and Orthopaedic
Surgery, Assistant Dean for Faculty Affairs,
Associate Director of Global REACH,
University of Michigan Medical School,
Ann Arbor, Michigan, USA

EDITOR

ASIF M. ILYAS, MD, FACS
Program Director of Hand Surgery, Professor
of Orthopaedic Surgery, Rothman Institute at
Jefferson, Philadelphia, Pennsylvania, USA

AUTHORS

IRFAN H. AHMED, MD
Assistant Professor, Department of
Orthopaedic Surgery, Rutgers New Jersey
Medical School, Newark, New Jersey, USA

**MUHAMMAD MUSTEHSAN BASHIR, FCPS
(Plastic Surgery), FCPS (Surgery)**
Associate Professor, Department of Plastic,
Reconstructive Surgery and Burn Unit, King
Edward Medical University, Mayo Hospital,
Lahore, Pakistan

GERARD CHANG, MD
Resident Physician, Rothman Institute at
Jefferson, Philadelphia, Pennsylvania, USA

TALIA R. CHAPMAN, MD
Department of Orthopaedic Surgery, Thomas
Jefferson University Hospitals, Philadelphia,
Pennsylvania, USA

NEAL C. CHEN, MD
Assistant Professor, Department of
Orthopaedic Surgery, Hand and Upper
Extremity Service, Massachusetts General
Hospital, Harvard Medical School, Boston,
Massachusetts, USA

KYLE R. EBERLIN, MD
Assistant Professor of Surgery, Division of
Plastic and Reconstructive Surgery, Associate
Director MGH Hand Surgery Fellowship,
Harvard Medical School, Massachusetts
General Hospital, Boston, Massachusetts,
USA

CARL M. HARPER, MD
Instructor, Department of Orthopaedics,
Beth Israel Deaconess Medical Center,
Harvard Medical School, Boston,
Massachusetts, USA

ASIF M. ILYAS, MD, FACS
Program Director of Hand Surgery,
Professor of Orthopaedic Surgery, Rothman
Institute at Jefferson, Philadelphia,
Pennsylvania, USA

MATTHEW L. IORIO, MD
Assistant Professor, Department of
Orthopaedics, Division of Plastic Surgery,
Beth Israel Deaconess Medical Center,
Harvard Medical School, Boston,
Massachusetts, USA

JUSTIN M. KISTLER, MD
Resident Physician, Orthopaedic Surgery,
Temple University Hospital, Philadelphia,
Pennsylvania, USA

CORY LEBOWITZ, DO
Department of Orthopedic Surgery, Rowan
University School of Osteopathic Medicine,
Stratford, New Jersey, USA

CHRISTOPHER J. LUCASTI, BS
Sidney Kimmel Medical College,
Philadelphia, Pennsylvania, USA

JONAS L. MATZON, MD
Associate Professor, Department of
Orthopaedic Surgery, Thomas Jefferson
University, Rothman Institute, Philadelphia,
Pennsylvania, USA

ANDREW MILLER, MD
Thomas Jefferson University Hospitals,
Philadelphia, Pennsylvania, USA

DAVID POPE, MD
Hand and Upper Extremity Surgery Fellow,
Department of Orthopaedic Surgery,
Allegheny General Hospital, Pittsburgh,
Pennsylvania, USA

TAMARA ROZENTAL, MD
Associate Professor, Department of
Orthopaedics, Beth Israel Deaconess
Medical Center, Harvard Medical School,
Boston, Massachusetts, USA

AARON J. RUBINSTEIN, MD
Resident Physician, Department of
Orthopaedic Surgery, Rutgers New Jersey
Medical School, Newark, New Jersey,
USA

HUSSAN BIRKHEZ SHAMI, MBBS
Postgraduate Resident, Department of Plastic,
Reconstructive Surgery and Burn Unit, King
Edward Medical University, Mayo Hospital,
Lahore, Pakistan

JONATHAN W. SHEARIN, MD
Hand and Upper Extremity Surgery,
Department of Orthopaedic Surgery,
Arnot Health, Elmira, New York, USA

**MUHAMMAD SOHAIL, FCPS (Plastic
Surgery), FCPS (Surgery)**
Assistant Professor, Department of Plastic,
Reconstructive Surgery and Burn Unit, King
Edward Medical University, Mayo Hospital,
Lahore, Pakistan

PETER TANG, MD, MPH, FAOA
Director, Center for Brachial Plexus and Nerve
Injury, Program Director, Hand and Upper
Extremity and Microvascular Surgery
Fellowship, Associate Professor, Department
of Orthopaedic Surgery, Allegheny General
Hospital, Drexel University College of
Medicine, Philadelphia, Pennsylvania, USA

JOSEPH J. THODER, MD
John W. Lachman Professor of Orthopaedic
Surgery and Sports Medicine, Lewis Katz
School of Medicine, Temple University,
Philadelphia, Pennsylvania, USA

BRIAN A. TINSLEY, MD
Hand Surgery Fellow, Rothman Institute at
Jefferson, Philadelphia, Pennsylvania, USA

RICK TOSTI, MD
Assistant Professor of Orthopaedic Surgery,
Philadelphia Hand to Shoulder Center, Sidney
Kimmel Medical College, Thomas Jefferson
University, Philadelphia, Pennsylvania, USA

JACOB E. TULIPAN, MD
Department of Orthopaedic Surgery, Thomas
Jefferson University, Philadelphia,
Pennsylvania

MICHAEL M. VOSBIKIAN, MD
Assistant Professor, Department of
Orthopaedic Surgery, Rutgers New Jersey
Medical School, Newark, New Jersey, USA

WILLIAM J. WARRENDER, MD
Department of Orthopaedic Surgery, Thomas
Jefferson University Hospitals, Philadelphia,
Pennsylvania, USA

Contents

Open fractures of the hand are a common and varied group of injuries. Although at increased risk for infection, open fractures of the hand are more resistant to infection than other open fractures. Numerous unique factors in the hand may play a role in the altered risk of postinjury infection. Current systems for the classification of open fractures fail to address the unique qualities of the hand. This article proposes a novel classification system for open fractures of the hand, taking into account the factors unique to the hand that affect its risk for developing infection after an open fracture.

Open fractures of the hand are thought to be less susceptible to infection than other open fractures because of the increased blood supply to the area. Current evidence for all open fractures shows that antibiotic use and the extent of contamination are predictive of infection risk but time to debridement is not. This article is a systematic review of the available literature on open fractures of the hand and upper extremity to determine infection rates based on the timing of debridement and antibiotic administration. The authors continue to recommend prompt debridement and treatment of most open fractures of the upper extremity.

Mangled hand injuries are defined as those with significant damage to multiple structures, which may be limb threatening. Historically, these injuries resulted in amputation or death, but modern surgical and perioperative advances allow for complex reconstruction and the possibility of a sensate and functional limb. Evaluation begins with surveying for life-threatening injuries followed by a systematic approach to identify injured structures; management begins with preserving all parts, minimizing warm ischemia time, performing debridement, and planning an operative approach to optimize the chance of a functional limb. With careful surgical planning and a well-executed reconstruction, most limbs can be salvaged.

Carpal tunnel syndrome (CTS) after distal radius fractures can present in 3 forms: acute, transient, and delayed. Acute CTS requires an emergent carpal tunnel release. Many patients with transient CTS after distal radius fracture do not require surgical release of the carpal tunnel once the fracture is repaired. Prophylactic carpal tunnel release in the absence of signs and symptoms of CTS after a distal radius fracture is not indicated. For patients with delayed CTS after a distal radius fracture, all possible causes of nerve compression should be considered and addressed in standard fashion.

Open distal radius fractures are rare injuries with few studies to guide treatment. The degree of soft tissue injury and contamination may be a primary consideration to dictate timing and operative intervention. Antibiotics should be started as early as possible and include a first-generation cephalosporin. Surgical fixation remains a matter of surgeon preference: although studies support the use of definitive internal fixation, many surgeons address contaminated injuries with external fixation. Although postoperative outcomes are similar to those of closed injuries for low-grade open distal radius fractures, high-grade injuries with more complex fracture patterns carry a high risk of complications, poor outcomes, and repeat surgical procedures.

Acute hand compartment syndrome is a potentially devastating condition a hand surgeon may be called on to evaluate and treat. This pathophysiologic cascade of events that begins with an inciting event progresses to increased intracompartmental pressure, tissue necrosis, and resultant morbidity and potentially mortality. Many patients present with an altered sensorium, making the diagnosis challenging, requiring the clinician to rely on clinical findings and intracompartmental pressure measurements. The timing to definitive treatment with complete decompressive fasciotomies is critical to optimize patient outcomes. The goals of treatment are to prevent contracture, functional disability, and the loss of limb or life.

Compartment syndrome of the forearm is uncommon but can have devastating consequences. Compartment syndrome is a result of osseofascial swelling leading to decreased tissue perfusion and tissue necrosis. There are numerous causes of forearm compartment syndrome, and high clinical suspicion must be maintained to avoid permanent disability. The most widely recognized symptoms include pain out of proportion and pain with passive stretch of the wrist and digits. Early diagnosis and decompressive fasciotomy are essential in the treatment of forearm compartment syndrome. Closure of fasciotomy wounds can often be accomplished by primary closure, but many patients require additional forms of soft tissue coverage procedures.

Soft tissue coverage of traumatic wounds of the upper extremity is often required to restore adequate function and form. An optimal coverage should be stable, durable, and able to withstand heavy demands of work, should allow free joint mobility, and should have an aesthetically acceptable appearance. Reconstructive options for coverage include autologous tissue and dermal skin substitutes. Multiple factors, including wound characteristics and complexity, general condition of the patient, and surgeon comfort and expertise, help in the selection of the reconstructive technique. This article summarizes commonly used soft tissue reconstructive options for traumatic wounds of the upper extremity.

The treatment goals of elbow fracture dislocations are congruent reduction of the ulnohumeral and radiocapitellar joints, stable fixation of the proximal ulna, stable fixation or arthroplasty of the radial head, and soft tissue repair. Fracture dislocations occur in patterns, and recognition of these patterns help guide surgical treatment. In patients with persistently unstable fractures after standard fixation, additional temporary joint spanning implants are useful to protect repairs.

Trauma to the upper extremity can present with an associated arterial injury. After patient stabilization, a thorough assessment with physical examination and various imaging modalities allows accurate diagnosis of the specific arterial injury. After diagnosis, efficient treatment is necessary to allow limb salvage. Treatment options include ligation, primary repair, graft reconstruction, endovascular repair, and amputation. The final treatment rendered is frequently dependent on injury location and mechanism. With any of the treatment options, complications may occur, including thrombosis. Currently, no validated anticoagulation protocol has been established for managing arterial injuries in the upper extremity.

Ulnar nerve dysfunction following distal humerus fractures is a well-recognized phenomenon. There is no consensus regarding the optimal handling of the ulnar nerve during surgical management of these fractures between in situ management and transposition. Using an electronic database to identify retrospective studies involving surgical fixation of distal humerus fractures yielded 46 studies, 5 trials meeting the authors' inclusion criteria, totaling 362 patients. An overall incidence of 19.3% for ulnar neuropathy was identified. Of those patients undergoing in situ release, the incidence was 15.3%. Of those who underwent transposition, there was a 23.5% incidence of ulnar neuropathy.

Radial nerve palsies are a common complication associated with humeral shaft fractures. The authors propose classifying these injuries into 4 types based on intraoperative findings: type 1, stretch/neuropraxia; type 2, incarcerated; type 3, partial transection; and type 4, complete transection. The initial management of radial nerve palsies associated with closed fractures of the humerus remains a controversial topic, with early exploration reserved for open fractures, fractures that cannot achieve an adequate closed reduction requiring fracture repair, fractures with associated vascular injuries, and patients with polytrauma. Outside of these recommendations, expectant observation for spontaneous recovery is recommended.

Patients who require assistive devices with their hands for mobilization are called functional quadrupeds. These patients pose a unique challenge after they have a distal radius fracture, as their injury not only limits the wrist but also compromises ambulation. The authors propose a different treatment strategy for functional quadrupeds to improve mobilization and weight bearing with the injured limb after a distal radius fracture. In this article, the authors define the functional quadruped and describe their technique of spanning bridge plate fixation with a retrospective review of patient outcomes.

HAND CLINICS

ISSUES OF RELATED INTEREST

Clinics in Sports Medicine, October 2014 (Vol. 33, No. 4)
Sports Injuries in the Military
Brett D. Owens, *Editor*
Available at: http://www.sportsmed.theclinics.com/

THE CLINICS ARE AVAILABLE ONLINE!
Access your subscription at:
www.theclinics.com

HAND CLINICS

Preface

Complex Trauma Management of the Upper Extremity

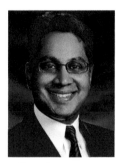

Asif M. Ilyas, MD, FACS
Editor

The hand and upper extremity are common sites of complex trauma. These injuries, be it from falls, motor vehicle accidents, industrial injuries, or ballistic or wartime trauma, can result in significant injuries resulting in not only injury to bones but also associated nerves, vessels, and the overlying skin. The upper extremity poses unique challenges with these complex injuries because of its unique anatomy requiring strong knowledge of the anatomy and intimate relationship between the neurovascular structures and skeletal anatomy. In this issue, we are fortunate to have leading surgeons of the upper extremity discussing management of these complex injuries.

The issue opens with a reexamination of open hand fractures and new ways to consider classifying them to better guide treatment. Antibiotic and surgical strategies are next examined, incorporating the best available evidence, followed by strategies to approach a mangled hand and upper extremity by utilizing a "damage control" approach. Compartment syndrome of the hand and forearm is also reviewed in detail.

The next area of focus is distal radius fractures, the most common fracture of the upper extremity treated surgically. This issue examines timing and surgical strategies for open distal radius fractures, and fracture management in the setting of polytrauma cases with bridge plating. Finally, carpal tunnel syndrome, a common complication of distal radius fractures, is also addressed relative to classification and surgical strategies.

Last, common soft tissue problems, including neurovascular injuries and traumatic wound management, are addressed. In particular, skin coverage strategies are discussed with particular attention to difficult areas, such as back of the hand and the posterior elbow. Common traumatic nerve injuries, including the ulnar nerve following distal humerus fractures and radial nerve injuries following humeral shaft fractures, are discussed. Controversy persists with how best to manage these nerve injuries, but evidence is presented and recommendations are made.

I am proud of the effort, writing, and guidance provided by the esteemed authors in this issue. I welcome comments and feedback as well as recommendations for future areas of analysis and study.

Asif M. Ilyas, MD, FACS
Rothman Institute at Thomas Jefferson University
925 Chestnut Street
Philadelphia, PA 19107, USA

E-mail address:
asif.ilyas@rothmaninstitute.com

Hand Clin 34 (2018) xi
https://doi.org/10.1016/j.hcl.2017.09.014
0749-0712/18/© 2017 Published by Elsevier Inc.

Open Fractures of the Hand
Review of Pathogenesis and Introduction of a New Classification System

Jacob E. Tulipan, MD*, Asif M. Ilyas, MD

KEYWORDS

• Open fractures • Hand • Pathogenesis • Classification system • Infection • Treatment

KEY POINTS

• Open fractures of the hand are commonly encountered, and vary widely in mechanism, location, and severity.
• Current evidence shows that antibiotic use and the extent of contamination are predictive of infection risk, but time to debridement is not.
• Open fractures of the hand are less susceptible to infection than other open fractures.
• The different regions of the hand are unique with regard to the osseous anatomy, blood supply, and soft tissue coverage, all of which factor into the risk of infection after an open fracture.
• Current classification schemas for open fractures are insufficient to describe and indicate treatment of fractures of the hand. A specialized classification is introduced that may better take into account risk factors for infection specific to the hand when determining best treatment of open fractures of the hand.

INTRODUCTION

Fractures of the finger, hand, and wrist constitute a significant disease burden, estimated to comprise up to 1.5% of emergency department visits and constituting 1.4 million cases in 1998 alone.[1] Like all fractures, distal upper extremity fractures range in severity based on several factors, including mechanism of injury, fracture location, fracture pattern, and associated soft tissue injury.

Open fractures of the hand are a common occurrence. A database study in 2001 estimated that 5% of hand fractures are open.[1] Like all open fractures, open hand and finger fractures are at increased risk for infection compared with their closed counterparts. Beginning with anecdotal observations that these fractures were less likely than other open fractures of the body to become infected, several studies have attempted to stratify these injuries by infection risk.

AVAILABLE EVIDENCE ON OPEN HAND FRACTURES

A study by McLain and colleagues[2] examined 208 consecutive patients with open fractures of the hand. Overall, the cohort showed an 11% infection rate. This study had limited subject retention (143 of 208 patients) and excluded both farm injuries and human bite wounds. All injuries were irrigated and debrided in the operating room and received cephalosporin plus/minus penicillin and an aminoglycoside preoperatively.

A similar retrospective analysis of factors correlating with infection in open hand fractures was performed by Swanson and colleagues.[3]

This article originally appeared in the January 2016 issue of *Orthopedic Clinics*, volume 47, issue 1.
Department of Orthopaedic Surgery, Thomas Jefferson University, 925 Chestnut Street, Philadelphia, PA 19107, USA
* Corresponding author. 1025 Walnut Street, Room 516 College, Philadelphia, PA 19107.
E-mail address: jacob.tulipan@gmail.com

hand.theclinics.com

These investigators showed a 6% incidence of infection in a series of 154 patients, with 35 lost to follow-up. As in the prior study, all patients were treated with prompt intravenous antibiotics and bedside or operative irrigation and debridement.

An in-depth analysis of functional recovery following open fractures in 75 patients performed by Duncan and colleagues[4] showed an infection rate of 6 per 171 fractures (3.5%), all in Gustilo-Anderson type III injuries. This group also underwent standard treatment with antibiotics and urgent irrigation and debridement.

More recent retrospective reviews have varied in the reported incidence of infection in open hand fracture. A 2011 review of 145 cases by Capo and colleagues[5] showed a 1.4% infection rate, even in a series with a high proportion (91 out of 145) of Gustilo-Anderson type III injuries. Similarly, a 2006 review of bone grafting for open fractures of the hand found a 0% infection rate even in more severe fractures.[6] Moreover, a 2010 retrospective review of 432 metacarpal and phalanx fractures requiring internal fixation found no significant difference in infection rates between the open (133 fractures) and closed (299 fractures) injury groups.[7]

These infection rates are significantly lower than that identified in a 2012 meta-analysis of all open fractures, not only hand open fractures, by Schenker and colleagues.[8] That review found an 8% infection rate in Gustilo-Anderson class I and II fractures, and a 12.7% rate in class III fractures. This finding supports the traditional wisdom that the hand is more resilient and less prone to infection after an open fracture than other open fractures of the body.

VARIABLES AFFECTING INFECTION RISK FOLLOWING AN OPEN FRACTURE OF THE HAND

There are several potential variables that may cause an open fracture to be more or less prone to developing an infection. These variables include the local osseous and soft tissue anatomy, the extent of contamination, the integrity of the soft tissue envelope, and the vascularity of the extremity.

Anatomy

Within the hand, distal to the radius and ulna, there are 27 bones that are prone to injury and an open fracture. Each has its unique anatomy, blood supply, and soft tissue coverage. Divided broadly, they can be separated into 3 regions: the phalanges, the metacarpals, and the carpal bones.

The soft tissue coverage of the phalanges consists of skin, tendon, ligament, areolar connective tissue, and nail. The 14 phalanges of each hand are devoid of muscle. As a result, the digits are prone to open injury with minimal amounts of trauma or fracture displacement, especially in the dorsal surface where the fascial layers lack the robustness of the palmar side. Furthermore, these structures do not possess the bulk or vascularity of muscle, potentially limiting their ability to fight infection.

The metacarpals share some morphologic features with the phalanges. Among these are palmar layers of tough fascia and alveolar connective tissue, and a dorsal surface with a thin covering of skin, tendon, and fascia. However, the metacarpals also benefit from the presence of interosseous, thenar, and hypothenar musculature, providing bulky coverage and blood supply. As a result, the metacarpals are vulnerable to dorsal open injuries and wounds but benefit from a robust blood supply.

The carpal bones possess the most dense soft tissue coverage of the osseous regions of the hand. However, they have the most fragile blood supply because of their absence of muscular coverage and otherwise extensive articular nature. Subsequently their blood supply is derived from their ligamentous and capsular attachments, structures that can be readily compromised with trauma. However, these soft tissue attachments, combined with the deep position of the carpus and its highly congruent and strong intercarpal attachments, provide resistance to open fractures in this region.

Vascular Supply

The digits receive most of their blood supply via the palmar digital arteries, with contribution from the dorsal digital arteries. Distally, these palmar arteries anastomose to form the blood supply to the digital pulp.[9] The palmar digital arteries run superficial to the digital nerves and lie directly deep to the skin. As a result of their position, these vessels are easily injured during digital trauma, compromising blood supply and increasing infection risk of the digit. This effect can be mitigated by the arterial anastomoses in the digit, which provide redundant blood supply in case of injury. Degloving, ring avulsion, and other circumferential injuries are a particular risk for dysvascularity, and loss of both radial and ulnar digital arteries can result in an avascular digit.

More proximally, the hand benefits from a robust and redundant vascularity. The vascular supply of the hand is provided by the palmar arches and variable dorsal arches, anastomotic networks composed of contributions from radial and ulnar circulation. These networks provide multiple perforators supplying both the metacarpal bones and the soft tissues surrounding them. The intrinsic muscles of the hand also possess multiple points of vascular supply, and provide a vascular bed that can supply the metacarpals. This region of the hand is more resistant to devascularization from trauma, although extensive soft tissue damage can still compromise its blood supply.

Proximal devascularization in hand injuries does not guarantee loss of blood supply distal to the injury. Although certain sites in the hand and wrist (eg, the proximal scaphoid) have tenuous vascular supply, the extensive network of anastomoses means that blood flow often has many alternate paths to reach distal structures. This supply is especially relevant to the carpus.

Because of the extensive articulations of the carpal bones, many have a limited, tenuous blood supply. A landmark study examining 75 cadaver limbs showed that the scaphoid received most of its blood supply via distal, dorsal nutrient vessels, with no intraosseous anastomosis to the palmar circulation. In 70% of capitates examined, most of the blood supply was dorsally based and did not anastomose with the palmar circulation. Likewise, in 8% of the lunate specimens examined, the vascular supply of the bone arose from a single vessel.[10]

Although the other carpal bones possess more redundant blood supply, all are vulnerable to disruption from high-energy injuries. In the case of the scaphoid and the capitate, in particular, small soft tissue disruptions may result in avascular bone stock, increasing the risk of infection and nonunion.

Severe vascular injuries of the hand may require emergent revascularization, regardless of the level of contamination of the wound. Although the literature is limited with regard to thrombosis and infection rate of revascularized hands in open fractures, inadequate perfusion necessitates emergent surgical intervention. Primary repair or grafting of damaged vessels prevents ischemic injury to distal structures, and must be performed if collateral circulation is not adequate. Poor blood supply is clearly a risk factor for subsequent infection.[11] However, the hand differs to some extent from other sites of open fracture in its extensive network of collateral circulation. Gustilo-Anderson type IIIc lower-limb fractures carry an infection risk as high as 39% according to one series.[12] However, there are limited data on infection rates in open hand injuries with vascular compromise.

Soft Tissue Envelope

The hand has a unique soft tissue envelope, both protective and potentially injurious in the setting of open hand fractures. The palmar surface of the hand benefits from a robust skin and dense subcutaneous tissue via its glabrous skin and deep fascial connections and muscular subcompartments. Significant trauma is required to result in open fractures on the palmar side. In contrast, the dorsal hand has only a thin layer of skin with minimal alveolar subcutaneous tissue, leaving the osseous and tendinous structures prone to ready exposure even with minor trauma.

When soft tissue loss is present, the hand poses a unique challenge in coverage. Securing adequate coverage in hand trauma is necessary to protect the deep osseous and soft tissue structures such as the many nerves, vessels, and tendons. However, many soft tissue coverage options exist that are indicated based on the nature of the injury and surgeon preference, including primary closure, secondary closure, acellular dermal substitutes, local rotational or advancement flaps, pedicled flaps, and free flaps. Each option has its own unique characteristics and risks and benefits for infection that must be taken into account in the setting of an open fracture.

Contamination

Frank contamination of an open fracture intuitively increases the risk for infection. Contamination of wounds often occurs as a result of injury mechanism, because debris is deposited into the wound site. These contaminant particles provide a nidus for bacterial growth, as well as serving as a source of bacterial bioburden. Certain types of contamination warrant specific consideration. Among these are soil contamination, which carries a high risk of anaerobic infection[13]; fecal contamination, which carries a risk of polymicrobial and gram-negative infection[14]; and bite wounds, which may be contaminated by organisms including *Eikenella* and *Pasteurella* species.[15] A 1978 study performed by Lawrence and colleagues[16] analyzed bacterial cultures of open fractures at time of presentation, and found that infections developed in a small proportion of patients (3 of 95 fractures), and only in those with high levels of contamination, providing evidence that initial degree of contamination affects infection risk.

Tscherne and Oestern[17] attempted to quantify this risk with their classification of open fractures. This classification takes into account the severity of associated soft tissue disruption, ranging from grade I (small puncture wound, negligible contamination, low-energy fracture) to grade III (heavy contamination, extensive soft tissue damage, associated neurovascular injury) and grade IV (traumatic amputation).[17] A 2015 retrospective review of 122 patients by Matos and colleagues[18] found that Tscherne II and III fractures were associated with a significantly higher rate of infection (48% and 26% respectively). Although this study examined both upper-limb and lower-limb injuries, it did not differentiate hand injuries specifically.

PREDICTIVE FACTORS IN OPEN HAND FRACTURES

A recent meta-analysis of 12 studies on open hand fractures meeting the inclusion criteria were reviewed to assess factors related to infection risk.[19] These factors included antibiotic administration and timing of debridement. Use of antibiotics varied between studies in the meta-analysis, but all studies using antibiotics used either a cephalosporin or a penicillin derivative. With all patients pooled, antibiotic use was significantly ($P = .0057$) associated with lower risk of infection, with a 4.4% infection rate in the antibiotic-treated group versus a 9.4% rate in the control group. Alternatively, timing to debridement was specifically examined in 2 of the studies used in the meta-analysis.[2,20] Neither study was able to show correlation between timing to debridement and infection rate, and nor did the pooled results.

Although not specific to the hand, several other studies have also examined open fractures of the distal radius and forearm, and studied different associated variables relative to infection risk.

A 2009 study by Glueck and colleagues[14] retrospectively reviewed 42 open distal radius fractures to determine infection risk. Three fractures ultimately became infected, of which 2 were grossly contaminated with fecal matter at the time of injury. Although the study found a statistically significant correlation between contamination and risk for infection, it failed to find any significant association between infection and either fixation method or time to debridement. All 3 infections occurred in Gustilo-Anderson type II or III injuries. These findings were mirrored in a 2011 study by Kurylo and colleagues,[21] which retrospectively identified 32 open radius fractures. This study failed to show any infections in the cohort, regardless of time to debridement or method of fixation. This study did not report degree of contamination.

A 2014 study by Zumsteg and colleagues[22] reviewed 200 open forearm fractures, and found a 5% infection rate. Deep infection risk was correlated with injury severity as measured by the Gustilo-Anderson classification, but was not associated with either time to debridement or time to

antibiotics. This study did not include information on the degree of contamination in these injuries.

The correlation between gross contamination and infection in the first study discussed earlier provides an indication that this is a significant contributor to infection risk. Although the distal radius differs from the hand in soft tissue coverage and vascularity, this association of injury characteristics and infection risk can be assumed to be analogous.

INAPPLICABILITY OF THE GUSTILO-ANDERSON CLASSIFICATION TO OPEN HAND FRACTURES

The Gustilo-Anderson classification[11,23] (Table 1), initially developed for use in long bones, is not optimal in classifying hand fractures. Specifically, the variables used to classify fractures in the Gustilo-Anderson system, particularly wound size, and the different nuances of soft tissue coverage and dysvascularity unique to the hand, make it less applicable to open hand fractures. For example, the laceration size cutoffs for Gustilo-Anderson types (1 cm and 10 cm) are not realistic for a limb as small as the hand and its fingers. In addition, the indications and options for soft tissue coverage of open long bone fractures (ie, Gustilo-Anderson type IIIB injuries) are very different in the hand. Furthermore, there are multiple common mechanisms for open fractures of the hand. The first is direct laceration or penetrating injury. In these cases, a sharp object (eg, a saw) cuts through skin and then the underlying soft

Table 1 The Gustilo-Anderson classification of open fractures	
Type	Description
I	Wound <1 cm
II	Wound >1 cm
IIIa	Extensive soft tissue laceration, wound >10 cm, adequate bone coverage, segmental fractures
IIIb	Inadequate soft tissue coverage over bone
IIIc	Arterial injury requiring repair

Data from Gustilo RB, Anderson JT. Prevention of infection in the treatment of one thousand and twenty-five open fractures of long bones: retrospective and prospective analyses. J Bone Joint Surg Am 1976;58(4):453–8; and Gustilo RB, Mendoza RM, Williams DN. Problems in the management of type III (severe) open fractures: a new classification of type III open fractures. J Trauma 1984;24(8):742–6.

Table 2 Proposed classification scheme for open fractures of the hand and fingers		
Type	**Location**	**Modifiers**
I II III	Phalanges Metacarpals Carpus	a: Primary soft tissue coverage not possible (**Fig. 1**) b: Frank contamination (**Fig. 2**) c: Dysvascularity requiring revascularization (**Fig. 3**)

tissues and bone. In the second mechanism, a crush injury tears skin while fracturing the bone below. In the third, shear forces avulse skin and break underlying bone. In addition, direct blows or falls can result in a bone spike being forcibly pushed through the skin. Each of these injuries can result in similar skin defects (and thus similar Gustilo-Anderson classes) while causing vastly different amounts of damage to the soft tissues and underlying bone.

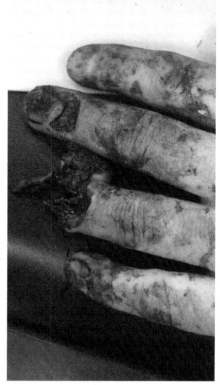

Fig. 2. A fracture showing frank contamination with soil. This fracture is classified as type Ib by the proposed classification scheme.

NEW CLASSIFICATION OF OPEN HAND FRACTURES

Given the current uncertainty with regard to risk factors for infection and appropriate timing to debridement of open fractures of the hand, we recommend the development of a new classification system to predict infection risk based on established risk factors for infection specifically after an open hand fracture. Subsequently, the classification system we are proposing (**Table 2**) deemphasizes wound size as the primary variable, and instead takes into account fracture location, extent of contamination, integrity of the soft tissue coverage, and viability of the vascularity.

By taking into account both anatomic and injury-specific factors, this classification can serve as a more effective tool for guiding treatment by providing insight for early infection risk stratification and long-term prognosis. We recommend using the classification in the following manner:

- Any open fracture type (I–III) without a modifier does not require emergent surgical treatment and can be managed with antibiotics and

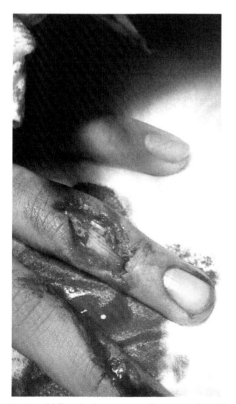

Fig. 1. A middle phalanx open fracture showing a soft tissue defect that cannot be closed primarily. This fracture is classified as type Ia by the proposed classification scheme.

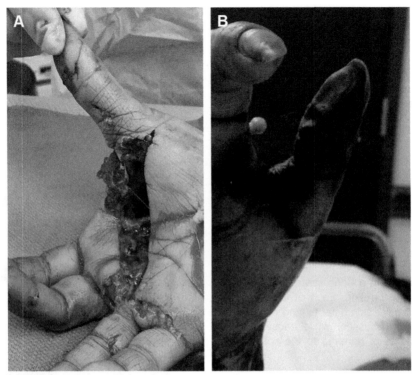

Fig. 3. An open fracture of the thumb and index metacarpal seen (*A*) immediately on presentation and (*B*) following open reduction and pinning without primary revascularization, showing late necrosis of avascular tissue. Although no direct vascular transection was evident, the traction and degloving nature of the injury resulted in late vascular compromise and subsequent infection. This fracture is classified as type IIc based on the proposed classification system and would have potentially benefited from early revascularization.

emergency room washout alone, followed by standard fracture management.

- Any open fracture type with the modifier "a" requires immediate antibiotics with emergency room washout alone, followed by semielective surgical soft tissue coverage and standard fracture management.
- Any open fracture type with the modifier "b" requires immediate antibiotics and urgent surgical debridement, followed by early versus delayed fracture management.
- Any open fracture type with the modifier "c" requires immediate antibiotics and emergent surgical revascularization and fracture management.

Using this system and algorithm has resulted in promising and consistent results in our patients. It is our expectation that with future research this open hand fracture–specific classification will be validated as a tool to help guide early treatment and prognose long-term outcome and infection risk more effectively than the currently used, nonspecific to hand, open fracture classifications.

REFERENCES

1. Chung KC, Spilson SV. The frequency and epidemiology of hand and forearm fractures in the United States. J Hand Surg 2001;26(5):908–15.
2. McLain RF, Steyers C, Stoddard M. Infections in open fractures of the hand. J Hand Surg 1991; 16(1):108–12.
3. Swanson TV, Szabo RM, Anderson DD. Open hand fractures: prognosis and classification. J Hand Surg 1991;16(1):101–7.
4. Duncan RW, Freeland AE, Jabaley ME, et al. Open hand fractures: an analysis of the recovery of active motion and of complications. J Hand Surg 1993; 18(3):387–94.
5. Capo JT, Hall M, Nourbakhsh A, et al. Initial management of open hand fractures in an emergency department. Am J Orthop 2011;40(12):E243–8.
6. Saint-Cyr M, Gupta A. Primary internal fixation and bone grafting for open fractures of the hand. Hand Clin 2006;22(3):317–27.
7. Bannasch H, Heermann AK, Iblher N, et al. Ten years stable internal fixation of metacarpal and phalangeal hand fractures-risk factor and outcome analysis show no increase of complications in the

treatment of open compared with closed fractures. J Trauma 2010;68(3):624–8.

8. Schenker ML, Yannascoli S, Baldwin KD, et al. Does timing to operative debridement affect infectious complications in open long-bone fractures? A systematic review. J Bone Joint Surg Am 2012;94(12): 1057–64.

9. Park HC, Bahar-Moni AS, Cho SH, et al. Classification of distal fingertip amputation based on the arterial system for replantation. J Hand Microsurg 2013; 5(1):4–8.

10. Gelberman RH, Gross MS. The vascularity of the wrist. Identification of arterial patterns at risk. Clin Orthop Relat Res 1986;(202):40–9.

11. Gustilo RB, Anderson JT. Prevention of infection in the treatment of one thousand and twenty-five open fractures of long bones: retrospective and prospective analyses. J Bone Joint Surg Am 1976; 58(4):453–8.

12. Soni A, Tzafetta K, Knight S, et al. Gustilo IIIC fractures in the lower limb: our 15-year experience. J Bone Joint Surg Br 2012;94(5):698–703.

13. Templeman DC, Gulli B, Tsukayama DT, et al. Update on the management of open fractures of the tibial shaft. Clin Orthop Relat Res 1998;(350):18–25.

14. Glueck DA, Charoglu CP, Lawton JN. Factors associated with infection following open distal radius fractures. Hand 2009;4(3):330–4.

15. Kennedy SA, Stoll LE, Lauder AS. Human and other mammalian bite injuries of the hand: evaluation and management. J Am Acad Orthop Surg 2015;23(1): 47–57.

16. Lawrence RM, Hoeprich PD, Huston AC, et al. Quantitative microbiology of traumatic orthopedic wounds. J Clin Microbiol 1978;8(6):673–5.

17. Tscherne H, Oestern HJ. A new classification of soft-tissue damage in open and closed fractures (author's transl). Unfallheilkunde 1982;85(3):111–5 [in German].

18. Matos MA, Lima LG, de Oliveira LA. Predisposing factors for early infection in patients with open fractures and proposal for a risk score. J Orthop Traumatol 2015;16(3):195–201.

19. Dwyer J, Ilyas A, Ketonis C. Timing of debridement and infection rates in open fractures of the hand: a systematic review. Journal of Hand Surgery 2014;39(9):e44.

20. Ng T, Unadkat J, Bilonick RA, et al. The importance of early operative treatment in open fractures of the fingers. Ann Plast Surg 2014;72(4):408–10.

21. Kurylo JC, Axelrad TW, Tornetta P III, et al. Open Fractures of the Distal Radius: The Effects of Delayed Debridement and Immediate Internal Fixation on Infection Rates and the Need for Secondary Procedures. Journal of Hand Surgery 2011;36(7):1131–4.

22. Zumsteg JW, Molina CS, Lee DH, et al. Factors influencing infection rates after open fractures of the radius and/or ulna. J Hand Surg 2014;39(5):956–61.

23. Gustilo RB, Mendoza RM, Williams DN. Problems in the management of type III (severe) open fractures: a new classification of type III open fractures. J Trauma 1984;24(8):742–6.

Antibiotic Management and Operative Debridement in Open Fractures of the Hand and Upper Extremity: A Systematic Review

William J. Warrender, MD[a], Christopher J. Lucasti, BS[b], Talia R. Chapman, MD[a], Asif M. Ilyas, MD[c],*

KEYWORDS

- Open fracture • Hand • Distal radius • Debridement • Antibiotics • Infection

KEY POINTS

- Infection rate for open fractures of the hand and upper extremity is low compared with open fractures of the lower extremity.
- Timing of operative debridement in open hand and upper extremity fractures has not been shown to consistently alter infection rates.
- Administration of antibiotics has been shown to lower infection rates in open fractures of the hand and upper extremity.
- We continue to recommend prompt, although not necessarily emergent, debridement and treatment of most open fractures of the upper extremity.

INTRODUCTION

Fractures of the hand and upper extremity constitute a significant disease burden in the United States. Finger, hand, and wrist fractures are estimated to comprise up to 1.5% of emergency department visits.[1] About 5% of these injuries are open fractures[1] and up to 11% of these can potentially become infected.[2] Like all open fractures, open upper extremity fractures are at increased risk for infection compared with their closed counterparts because of the associated soft tissue injury and contamination of deep structures. Existing literature on open fracture infection rates and treatment guidelines have focused primarily on the lower extremity, with limited guidelines available for the upper extremity.

Open fractures of the hand are thought to be less susceptible to infection than other open fractures likely because of the increased blood supply to the area.[2,3] Also, upper extremity injuries of the hand are more amenable to local analgesia than lower extremity injuries thereby facilitating earlier bedside debridement and washout. Current evidence for all open fractures shows that antibiotic use and the extent of contamination are predictive of infection risk, but time to debridement is not.[4] With this in mind, is it still necessary to take the

Disclosure Statement: The authors have no financial interests in any of the products or techniques mentioned and have received no external support related to this study.

[a] Department of Orthopaedic Surgery, Thomas Jefferson University Hospital, Philadelphia, PA, USA; [b] Sidney Kimmel Medical College, Philadelphia, PA, USA; [c] Rothman Institute, Thomas Jefferson University, 925 Chestnut Street, Philadelphia, PA 19107, USA

* Corresponding author.

E-mail address: asif.ilyas@rothmaninstitute.com

patient with an open upper extremity fracture to the operating room as urgently as a lower extremity fracture? And if so, in what circumstances? To guide management, we reviewed the available literature on open fractures of the hand and upper extremity to determine infection rates, based on the timing of debridement and antibiotic administration.

METHODS

A comprehensive literature review was performed to identify all studies on antibiotic management and timing to debridement after open fractures of the upper extremity. Searches for the terms "open fracture" and "upper extremity," "phalangeal," "hand," "distal radius," "forearm," "elbow," "humerus," and "shoulder" were performed using the search engines PubMed, Medline, Google Scholar, UpToDate, Cochrane Reviews, CINAHL, and Scopus (from inception to October 2016). Reference sections of relevant articles were reviewed to identify further relevant trials. Inclusion criteria for our systematic review were all studies (level I-V) that reported on infections rates in upper extremity fractures related to antibiotic protocols and timing of debridement. Studies that included lower extremity open fractures were only included if they also involved relevant open fractures of the upper extremity. Exclusion criteria were non–English language articles, nonhuman studies, retracted papers, and studies that did not comment on infection rates. Preferred Reporting Items for Systematic Reviews and Meta-Analyses (PRISMA) criteria were followed throughout the study. Data were abstracted in duplicate by two authors (WJW, CJL).

RESULTS

A combined total of 14 studies met our inclusion criteria. A PRISMA flow diagram is found in **Fig. 1**, detailing our literature search, with included and excluded studies. Results are reports by anatomic area and subdivided by antibiotic management and timing of operative debridement.

OPEN HAND FRACTURES
Antibiotic Management

Routine use of antibiotics in managing open fractures of the fingers and hand is not consistent between providers as with open fractures of other long bones (**Table 1**). There is a noticeable paucity of objective literature to either support or refute their importance. Sloan and colleagues[5] analyzed distal phalangeal fractures prospectively and found a 30% increase in the incidence of infection

when antibiotics were not used. Patients were randomly allocated to one of four treatment groups: (1) no antibiotics; (2) cephradine (a first-generation cephalosporin), 500 mg orally four times a day for 5 days; (3) cephradine, 1 g intravenously preoperatively and then 500 mg orally four times a day for 5 days; or (4) cephradine, I g intravenously preoperatively and I g orally postoperatively. After the first 40 patients were enrolled, three proven cases of infection had occurred, all of which were in the no antibiotic group. There was a significantly higher infection rate than for those treated with antibiotics ($P = .02$) and it was believed that it would be unethical to continue this group. No difference between remaining groups treated with antibiotics was found to be significant. Similarly, Ng and colleagues[6] performed a retrospective review that included 70 patients with open fractures of the hand and found that there was a significant difference between infection rates of those who received and did not receive intravenous antibiotics ($P = .0072$). Administration of intravenous antibiotics in the emergency department was the most significant factor in preventing infection. Intravenous antibiotics were administered early (authors report "in the emergency room" but no specific time frame) in 53 (75.7%) patients. Seventy-seven percent of these patients were given intravenous 1 to 2 g of cefazolin. Five patients received 600 mg of clindamycin, three received 100 mg of gentamicin, and four patients received the antibiotics at an outside hospital and therefore did not have documentation as to the type or dosage. The overall infection rate was 11.4%. Additionally, a more recent meta-analysis reporting on infection risk in open hand fractures found that with all patients pooled, antibiotic use was significantly ($P = .0057$) associated with lower risk of infection, with a 4.4% infection rate in the antibiotic group versus a 9.4% rate in the control group.[7] Use of antibiotics varied between studies in the meta-analysis, but all studies using antibiotics used either a cephalosporin or a penicillin derivative.[8] Finally, Capo and colleagues[8] also support early antibiotic administration. They reported an infection rate of 1.4% following a study of 145 cases of open hand fractures with a mean delay of less than 4 hours from injury to first antibiotics administration. The two patients that developed infections were successfully managed with a 5-day course of cephalexin.

However, after a prospective trial including 91 operatively treated open phalangeal fractures, Suprock and colleagues[9] reported no difference in infection rate with early use of oral antibiotics in fractures that have been aggressively irrigated

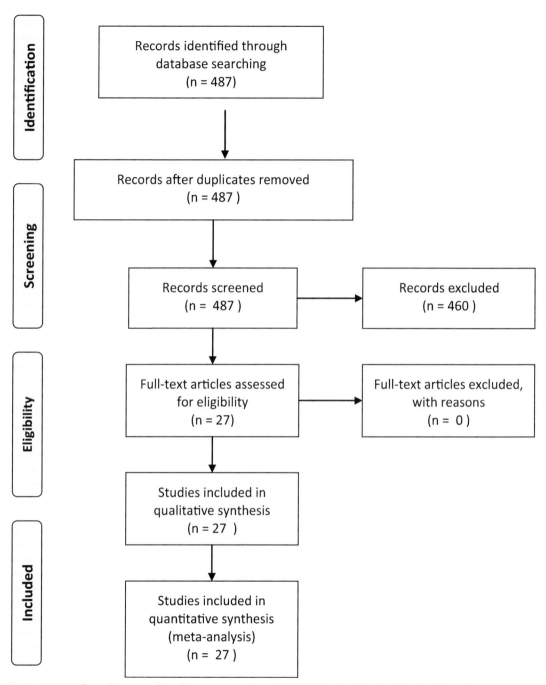

Fig. 1. PRISMA flow diagram of the literature search, which includes included and excluded studies.

and debrided compared with patients treated with aggressive irrigation and debridement alone. Their antibiotic regimen was a first-generation cephalosporin, dicloxacillin or erythromycin orally for 3 days. The authors conclude that antibiotics should not be routinely used in the treatment of open finger fractures, but may play a role in helping prevent infections of the fingers in patients who have significant amounts of devitalized tissue or who are noncompliant in follow-up care.

Timing of Debridement

With regards to the importance of timing of debridement in open fracture of the hand, a study by McLain and colleagues[10] examined 208

Table 1
Antibiotic management

Reference	Location of Fracture	Noninfection		Infection		P Values (Early vs Late Debridement)	Total
		Early Debridement (<8 h)	Late or No Debridement (>8 h)	Early Debridement (<8 h)	Late or No Debridement (>8 h)		
McLain et al,[10] 1991	Hand	127	0	16 (11%)	0	—	143
Swanson et al,[11] 1991	Hand	147	0	5	2	—	154
Zumsteg et al,[12] 2014	Forearm	28	162	2 (7%)	8 (5%)	.6500	200
Glueck et al,[13] 2009	Distal radius	0	39	3 (7%)	0	—	42
Kurylo et al,[14] 2011	Radius	0	32	0	0	—	32
MacKay et al,[15] 2013	Distal radius	599	0	2	0	—	601
Yang and Eisler,[16] 2003	Distal radius	0	12	0	0	—	12
Malhotra et al,[17] 2014	Upper extremity	87	26	13 (13%)	3 (10%)	>.9900	129
Total		988	271	41	13	—	1313

consecutive patients with open fractures of the hand and report that treatment delay had no effect on the incidence of infection (**Table 2**). The average delay from injury to debridement for wounds that became infected was 6.9 hours and for noninfected wounds it was 7.3 hours. No infections occurred in patients treated more than 12 hours after injury, and many patients who developed infections received treatment earlier than those who did not develop infection. Seventy-five percent of all patients had wounds debrided within 8 hours of injury and 95% within 16 hours. Overall, the cohort showed an 11% infection rate. Of note, the study had poor subject retention (143 of 208 patients) and excluded farm injuries and human bite wounds. All injuries were irrigated and debrided in the operating room and received cephalosporin with or without penicillin and an aminoglycoside. Along the same line, Ng and colleagues[6] report that the timing of debridement did not predict infection and washout in the emergency department was not significantly related to infection ($P = .73$). Mean time to surgery was 2.3 hours with an overall infection rate of 11.4%. Timing to debridement was specifically examined in two of the studies in the previously mentioned meta-analysis.[7] Neither study was able to show correlation between timing to debridement and infection rate, nor did the pooled results. Among these, Capo and colleagues[8] report the mean delay from injury to debridement in the emergency department was less than 6 hours and concluded that delayed surgical management is not associated with a higher infection rate.

Conversely, one study by Swanson and colleagues[11] reported on a retrospective analysis of factors correlating with infection in open hand fractures. Two of their seven patients in whom infections developed had a delay in treatment greater than 24 hours, although they do not describe the nature of this delay. Overall they had a 6% incidence of infection in 154 patients with 35 lost to follow-up.

OPEN DISTAL RADIUS AND FOREARM FRACTURES
Antibiotic Management

A 2014 study by Zumsteg and colleagues[12] reviewed 200 open forearm fractures and reported a 5% infection rate (see **Table 1**). Deep infection risk was not associated with time to antibiotics. The average time to antibiotic administration was not significantly different in patients developing deep infection or nonunion. There was also no significant difference in the rates of deep infection or nonunion in patients receiving antibiotics in less

than 3 hours compared with those who did not. Patients with Gustilo-Anderson type 1 and 2 fractures received 2-g cefazolin, and patients with type 3 fractures received 1-g vancomycin in combination with 750-mg levofloxacin. Patients with penicillin allergies were provided with either 2-g aztreonam or 900-mg clindamycin as a substitute.[12]

Timing of Debridement

Glueck and colleagues[13] report that time to debridement was not a significant predictor of infection in open distal radius fractures (see **Table 2**). They report three (7%) total infections in 42 patients that were followed for an average of 15 months. In their three infected cases, time to debridement averaged 6 hours, which is less than the average time to debridement in the study of 7.7 hours. Of note, two of the three infections were grossly contaminated with fecal matter at the time of injury. All three infections occurred in Gustilo-Anderson type II or III injuries. Although the study found a statistically significant correlation between contamination and risk for infection, they found no relationship between infection and time to initial irrigation and debridement, method of fixation, Gustilo-Anderson type, or Swanson type.[13]

These findings were echoed in a 2011 study by Kurylo and colleagues.[14] They retrospectively identified 32 open radius fractures and failed to show any infections in the cohort, regardless of time to debridement. The average time from arrival at the hospital to the operating room was 15 hours, 4 minutes. The reasons for delay included the need for medical stabilization for nine patients and a shortage of operating room space in 11 instances. No patient developed an infection through the time of their last follow-up, with an average follow-up of 34 weeks reported.

Similarly, MacKay and coworkers[15] compared open distal radius fractures treated with early debridement and fixation with individually matched closed fractures treated operatively with greater than 1 year of follow-up, and identified a similar infection rate in both groups. There was one pin tract infection in each group, both successfully treated with oral antibiotics of the 601 patients with a distal radius fracture. Patients who sustained an open fracture received tetanus, intravenous antibiotics, reduction, sterile dressing application, and splinting in the emergency department. All open fractures underwent irrigation, debridement, and operative fixation within 24 hours of presentation with average time of 8.1 hours and a range of 3 to 22 hours.

Table 2
Timing of debridement

Reference	Location of Fracture	Noninfection		Infection		P Values (Antibiotics vs Late or No Antibiotics)	Total
		Antibiotics/Early Administration	No Antibiotics/Late Administration	Antibiotics/Early Administration	No Antibiotics/Late Administration		
Sloan et al,[5] 1987	Distal phalangeal	71	7	2 (2.8%)	3 (30%)	.0200	83
Ng et al,[6] 2014	Hand	53	9	0	8	.0072	70
Ketonis et al,[7] 2017	Hand	1330	155	61 (4.4%)	16 (9.4%)	.0057	1669
Capo et al,[8] 2011	Hand	143	0	2 (1.4%)	0	—	145
Suprock et al,[9] 1990	Phalangeal	43	44	2 (2.1%)	2 (2.1%)	—	91
Zumsteg et al,[12] 2014	Forearm	150	40	9 (6%)	1 (2%)	.4000	200
Total		1790	255	76	30	—	2258

Zumsteg and colleagues[12] reviewed 200 open forearm fractures, and also found that deep infection risk was not associated with time to debridement. Specifically, there were no significant differences in the rates of deep infection or nonunion in patients undergoing debridement in fewer than 6 hours, compared with those who did not. Their overall infection rate was 5%. Deep infection developed at a mean of 118 days after initial fixation. Three infections developed within the first 30 days, whereas the remaining seven developed at more than 90 days after initial fixation.[12] Finally, Yang and Eisler[16] evaluated the timing of surgical debridement for 91 grade one open fractures at various sites, including lower extremity fractures. The 12 patients with open distal radius fractures had no infections or nonunions even though all patients were debrided more than 12 hours after injury.[16]

UPPER EXTREMITY FRACTURES (UNSPECIFIED)
Timing of Debridement

Malhotra and colleagues[17] evaluated the rates of deep infections of open fractures in relation to the time to the first irrigation and debridement (see **Table 2**). In the upper extremity, there was no significant difference if the irrigation and debridement was delayed (<8 hours, 13% vs >8 hours, 10%; P>.99). All patients received appropriate prophylactic antimicrobials. In the upper extremity, only higher Gustilo-Anderson type correlated with the incidence of infection. In contrast, delay of greater than 8 hours to first debridement for open fractures of the lower extremity increased the likelihood of infection.

DISCUSSION

The current literature indicates that the overall infection rate for open fractures of the upper extremity is low and that there is a correlation between the administration of antibiotics and lower infection rates.[5–18] Unfortunately, because of the broad range of antibiotic regimens used in the literature, we are unable to recommend a regimen that is optimal for any particular fracture pattern. In the hand, oral antibiotics are likely sufficient with intravenous regimens being reserved for severe soft tissue injury and contamination. Patients with open distal radius fractures should receive antibiotics but the timing of the antibiotics does not correlate with risk of infection. It is also advisable to become familiar with the community methicillin-resistant *Staphylococcus aureus* prevalence in one's area to help tailor antibiotic

coverage.[19,20] The use of antibiotics in the treatment of open fractures of the long bones is widely accepted as standard of care and their effectiveness has been proven in random prospective studies by Patzakis and colleagues[21] and Gustilo and Anderson.[22]

Based on our review and the available data, timing of debridement in open upper extremity fractures has not been shown to alter infection rates. The timing of debridement for open hand and upper extremity fractures is less important than administration of antibiotics. Our review suggests that early debridement (<8 hours) of open hand and upper extremity fractures has not been shown to effect infection rates.[5–18] This is in contrast to open fractures of the lower extremity according to Malhotra and colleagues.[17] Delay of greater than 8 hours to first debridement for open fractures of the lower extremity increased the likelihood of infection (<8 hours, 10% vs >8 hours, 27%; P = .002). Interestingly, the overall rates of infection for the upper (12%) and lower (12%) extremities were similar (P>.99).

The treatment and prognosis of open upper extremity fractures is distinct from that of open long bone fractures. Some believe and have proposed that the low incidence of infections after open fractures of the hand and upper extremity is because of its robust blood supply.[22–24] Even the most severe hand injuries requiring replantation have a much lower infection rate (approximately 1% to 2% after digital replantation) than open long bone fractures.[25–27] This finding supports the traditional wisdom that the hand is more resilient and less prone to infection after an open fractures of the lower extremity.

A specialized classification was recently introduced by Tulipan and Ilyas[3] that may better take into account risk factors for infection specific to the hand when determining best treatment of open fractures of the hand. Instead of focusing on the size of the wound associated with an open fracture, this classification system strives to be more prognostic and guide treatment by weighing an open hand fracture's anatomic location, associated soft tissue injury, and extent of contamination.

Our study faced some limitations. Like with any systematic review of meta-analysis, the findings are based on and limited to the available data. Moreover, the findings may be confounded by the varied study protocols used. In addition, studies involving open fractures were found to be highly variable in terms of the technique and thoroughness of the "debridement." Similarly, the degree of contamination was not consistently recorded or qualified. Anatomically, there are more studies available regarding open hand fractures as compared with open distal radius fractures and other more proximal open upper extremity fractures. Ideally, future studies should consider multicenter prospective designs, with preferable randomization of treatment techniques. However, the highly variable nature of open fractures and the acuity of its management makes such studies difficult to perform.

SUMMARY

The timing of debridement for open hand and upper extremity fractures is less important than the timely administration of antibiotics with open hand and upper extremity fractures in improving infection risk.[5–18] We continue to support prompt, although not necessarily emergent, debridement and treatment of most open fractures of the upper extremity, recognizing that each patient's clinical situation must be considered individually. Overall, the infection rate for open fractures of the hand and upper extremity is low.[5–18]

REFERENCES

1. Chung KC, Spilson SV. The frequency and epidemiology of hand and forearm fractures in the United States. J Hand Surg 2001;26(5):908–15.
2. Roth AI, Fry DE, Polk HC. Infectious morbidity in extremity fractures. J Trauma 1986;26(8):757–61.
3. Tulipan JE, Ilyas AM. Open fractures of the hand: review of pathogenesis and introduction of a new classification system. Orthop Clin North Am 2016;47(1):245–51.
4. Schenker ML, Yannascoli S, Baldwin KD, et al. Does timing to operative debridement affect infectious complications in open long-bone fractures? A systematic review. J Bone Joint Surg Am 2012;94(12):1057–64.
5. Sloan JP, Dove AF, Maheson M, et al. Antibiotics in open fractures of the distal phalanx? J Hand Surg Br 1987;12(1):123–4.
6. Ng T, Unadkat J, Bilonick RA, et al. The importance of early operative treatment in open fractures of the fingers. Ann Plast Surg 2014;72(4):408–10.
7. Ketonis C, Dwyer J, Ilyas AM. Timing of debridement and infection rates in open fractures of the hand: a systematic review. Hand 2017;12(2):119–26.
8. Capo JT, Hall M, Nourbakhsh A, et al. Initial management of open hand fractures in an emergency department. Am J Orthop 2011;40(12):E243–8.
9. Suprock MD, Hood JM, Lubahn JD. Role of antibiotics in open fractures of the finger. J Hand Surg Am 1990;15(5):761–4.
10. McLain RF, Steyers C, Stoddard M. Infections in open fractures of the hand. J Hand Surg Am 1991;16(1):108–12.
11. Swanson TV, Szabo RM, Anderson DD. Open hand fractures: prognosis and classification. J Hand Surg Am 1991;16(1):101–7.
12. Zumsteg JW, Molina CS, Lee DH, et al. Factors influencing infection rates after open fractures of the radius and/or ulna. J Hand Surg Am 2014;39(5):956–61.
13. Glueck DA, Charoglu CP, Lawton JN. Factors associated with infection following open distal radius fractures. Hand (N Y) 2009;4(3):330–4.
14. Kurylo JC, Axelrad TW, Tornetta P, et al. Open fractures of the distal radius: the effects of delayed debridement and immediate internal fixation on infection rates and the need for secondary procedures. J Hand Surg 2011;36(7):1131–4.
15. MacKay BJ, Montero N, Paksima N, et al. Outcomes following operative treatment of open fractures of the distal radius: a case control study. Iowa Orthop J 2013;33:12–8.
16. Yang EC, Eisler J. Treatment of isolated type I open fractures: is emergent operative debridement necessary? Clin Orthop Relat Res 2003;410:289–94.
17. Malhotra AK, Goldberg S, Graham J, et al. Open extremity fractures: impact of delay in operative debridement and irrigation. J Trauma Acute Care Surg 2014;76(5):1201–7.
18. Rozental TD, Beredjiklian PK, Steinberg DR, et al. Open fractures of the distal radius. J Hand Surg Am 2002;27(1):77–85.
19. Centers for Disease Control and Prevention. 2014. Active bacterial core surveillance report, emerging infections program network, methicillin-resistant staphylococcus aureus, 2014.
20. Sakoulas G, Moellering RC. Increasing antibiotic resistance among methicillin-resistant Staphylococcus aureus strains. Clin Infect Dis 2008;46(Suppl 5):S360–7.
21. Patzakis MJ, Harvey JP, Ivler D. The role of antibiotics in the management of open fractures. J Bone Joint Surg Am 1974;56(3):532–41.
22. Gustilo RB, Anderson JT. Prevention of infection in the treatment of one thousand and twenty-five open fractures of long bones: retrospective and prospective analyses. J Bone Joint Surg Am 1976;58(4):453–8.
23. Gingrass RP, Fehring B, Matloub H. Intraosseous wiring of complex hand fractures. Plast Reconstr Surg 1980;66(3):383–94.
24. Granberry WM. Gunshot wounds of the hand. Hand 1973;5(3):220–8.
25. Szabo RM, Spiegel JD. Infected fractures of the hand and wrist. Hand Clin 1988;4:477–89.
26. Morrison WA, O'Brien BM, MacLeod AM. Evaluation of digital replantation: a review of 100 cases. Orthop Clin North Am 1977;8(2):295–308.
27. Tamai S. Twenty years' experience of limb replantation: review of 293 upper extremity replants. J Hand Surg Am 1982;7(6):549–56.

"Damage Control" Hand Surgery
Evaluation and Emergency Management of the Mangled Hand

Rick Tosti, MD[a], Kyle R. Eberlin, MD[b],*

KEYWORDS

- Hand Injuries • Mangled Hand • Hand Reconstruction • Hand Amputation

KEY POINTS

- Mangled hand injuries are defined as those with significant damage to multiple structures, which threatens the function and/or viability of the limb.
- The mantra, "life before limb," or a decision to salvage versus amputate must be considered, taking in the overall injury burden when determining surgical options that are best for patients, short term and long term.
- Excessive time without perfusion of the amputated part can lead to irreversible tissue necrosis. Tissue necrosis can at times be obviated if the part is preserved in a cool environment. If ischemia time allows, a common order of fixation includes bone, extensor tendon, flexor tendon, artery, nerve, vein, and skin.
- Post-revascularization, a warm environment (warm room, heating device such as a warming blanket, or both), daily aspirin for 1 month, and intravenous antibiotics for 3 days are recommended.
- Post-revascularization, additional procedures are routine and patients should be prepared in advance for their need.

INTRODUCTION

Mangled hand injuries are defined as those with significant damage to multiple structures, which threatens the function and/or viability of the limb. Historically, these injuries resulted in death or amputation, but with modern advances in débridement, antibiotics, skeletal fixation, microsurgery, and soft tissue coverage, successful and functional reconstruction of a severely damaged limb is possible.[1] The injury mechanisms resulting in mangling injuries generally are high energy and include either a sharp laceration or a crush/avulsion force. Concomitant disruption of skin, nerves, vessels, bones, joints, tendons, and muscles presents a challenging clinical situation to treating surgeons, who must decide between salvage and amputation. Fortunately, mangling upper extremity injuries are uncommon; only 5% of all

Conflict of Interest Statement: Each author certifies that he or she has no commercial associations (eg, consultancies, stock ownership, equity interest, patent/licensing arrangements, etc) that might pose a conflict of interest in connection with the submitted article.

Location Statement: Research for this article was conducted at Massachusetts General Hospital, Boston, MA.

[a] Department of Orthopedic Surgery, The Philadelphia Hand Center, Sidney Kimmel Medical College, Thomas Jefferson University, 834 Chestnut Street Suite G114, Philadelphia, PA 19107, USA; [b] Division of Plastic and Reconstructive Surgery, Harvard Medical School, Massachusetts General Hospital, Wang Building, 55 Fruit Street, Boston, MA 02114, USA

* Corresponding author.

E-mail address: keberlin@mgh.harvard.edu

Hand Clin 34 (2018) 17–26

https://doi.org/10.1016/j.hcl.2017.09.002

hand fractures are open and a vast majority of injuries are not limb threatening.[2] As a result of its rarity, however, many trauma centers, including those with American College of Surgeons trauma designation, are not equipped to treat these injuries.

Paramount to treatment of the mangled hand is the mantra, "life before limb." The decision for salvage versus amputation can be difficult; surgeons must consider the overall injury burden and are obligated to consider all options for surgical reconstruction, including the possibility of amputation with prosthetic use. This article discusses the evaluation of the mangled limb, perioperative management strategies, and outcomes.

INITIAL EVALUATION AND EMERGENCY MANAGEMENT

A patient's first encounter with a health care provider is either at the site of injury or in an emergency department. Depending on the severity of the trauma burden, patients may require standard Advanced Trauma Life Support. In general, the authors recommend against the routine use of tourniquet in the field unless direct pressure does not provide sufficient hemostasis, which is rare.

Appropriate preservation of the amputated or dysvascular extremity is critical. Excessive time without perfusion can lead to irreversible tissue necrosis. Tissue necrosis can at times be obviated if the part is preserved in a cool environment. The authors recommend washing the part to remove debris, then wrapping it in moist gauze. The part is then placed into a plastic bag or container and then placed into another plastic bag filled with ice. Avoid placing the part directly on ice, because frostbite may cause irrevocable injury. The generally accepted limits of warm ischemia are 12 hours for a digit and 6 hours for a more proximal injury,[1] although these are not absolute. Proximal injuries have less tolerance for ischemia due to the higher metabolic requirements of muscle. The ischemic time limits can be doubled for a cooled, well-preserved part.[3] Replantation has been successfully performed as late as 94 hours for a digit and 54 hours for a hand when appropriately preserved.[4,5]

On arrival to the hospital, a few simple steps can greatly assist the treating surgeon and expedite the process of care (**Box 1**). If an upper arm tourniquet is present, it is removed carefully with an understanding of the total ischemia time, patient comorbidities (specifically coronary artery disease and regularity of cardiac rhythm), and the risk of a potassium bolus with reperfusion. Often, the wound is already hemostatic because thrombus

---

Box 1
Tips for the emergency physician

Mind the airway, breathing, circulation (ABCs) first

Hold firm, focused pressure on bleeding wounds first before applying a tourniquet

Note pertinent history information

Perform a focused physical examination

Carefully note vascular status and place pulse oximeter on all affected digits

Administer antibiotics

Inquire tetanus status and treat appropriately

Irrigate the wound and remove debris

Cover and splint the limb

Obtain radiographs and include amputated part within radiographic field

Ensure the amputated part is properly preserved

---

has formed at the site of arterial injury. If hemostasis is not controlled, then the authors recommend holding pressure (ideally a single finger over the bleeding vessel) for 10 minutes to control bleeding. A pressure dressing also may be applied. If all techniques fail, then the tourniquet can be replaced knowing that swift transition to the operating room is crucial.

A hand and upper extremity surgeon is usually consulted in an urgent fashion for mangled injuries of the hand. If the patient is awake, the surgeon should take a history noting pertinent items related to surgical decision making: age, hand dominance, mechanism of injury, time of injury, comorbidities, medications, occupation, smoking status, tetanus status, method of preserving the amputated part, and patient preferences. Physical examination should include inspection noting deformity and the size, depth, and trajectory of each wound. Palpation can determine the stability of the skeleton and the joints. The patient should then be asked to actively move the affected limb and the digits, which gives insight into nerve, muscle, and tendon function. If the patient cannot move the digits, then using the tenodesis effect (noting extension of the fingers with passive wrist flexion and noting flexion of the fingers with passive wrist extension) can be helpful in determining the integrity of the tendons. A sensory examination should be performed with careful 2-point discrimination in all nerve distributions.

With mangled hands, the vascular examination is critically important. The surgeon should observe the color of the limb and palpate the digits for temperature and turgor. Capillary refill should be 2 or 3 seconds. Brachial, radial, and ulnar pulses are palpated and graded for strength. If no pulse is present, a Doppler ultrasound should also be used and the palmar arch and the digital arteries should be auscultated. If the perfusion seems inadequate, a pulse oximeter should be placed on the digit; a reading higher than 95% with a pulsatile waveform confirms that the digit is perfused.[6] The authors do not recommend pricking the finger with a needle to observe bleeding; multiple pricks or large bore needles can cause discoloration and/or disrupt critical microcirculation at the tip.

Adjunct laboratory and imaging tests are commonly performed; a complete blood cell count and basic metabolic profile with coagulation parameters are helpful. Radiographs are most useful after the limb has been reasonably aligned (traction view). The amputated part, if present, should also be filmed in the same radiographic field to allow for easy viewing intraoperatively. CT scan can assist surgical planning of fractures but is often not necessary or possible when operative intervention is undertaken emergently.

OPERATIVE MANAGEMENT

Operative intervention should proceed immediately for a threatened limb. Antibiotics are administered as soon as possible; the authors typically use a first-generation cephalosporin to cover gram-positive bacteria and gentamicin (5 mg/kg every 24 hours) for gram-negative coverage. Penicillin (2–4 million units) is added to prevent clostridium infection if farm or soil contamination is present.

Major limb surgery can be lengthy and complicated; thoughtful preoperative discussion with the surgical and anesthetic team is important regarding the equipment, placement of Foley catheter, patient positioning, use of a leg drape if needed for donor veins and nerves, and anticipated length of surgery. For procedures involving revascularization, the authors prefer placement of a preoperative indwelling catheter to promote vasodilation and assist with postoperative pain. A back table can be invaluable in the setting of amputated parts; it is most efficient to begin identifying and labeling structures on the amputated part at the back table while the remainder of the anesthesia and surgical team is preparing the patient (**Fig. 1**).

The first step in treating a mangled extremity is to carefully assess the damaged structures in a systematic, organized way. The surgeon should be careful not to sacrifice small skin bridges, which

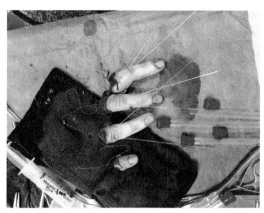

Fig. 1. A sterile back table can be useful in improving the efficiency of surgery. In this patient, all 4 fingers underwent débridement, identification of structures, suturing of tendons, bone shortening, and preloaded Kirschner wire fixation. All of this was completed while the operating team was preparing the room and patient.

may contain intact critical veins for drainage. Large-volume irrigation should be used to remove loose debris, and all devitalized tissue should be sharply removed. Deflating the tourniquet and observing tissue perfusion may assist in determining the viability of tissues. For the skin and soft tissues, this may require resecting skin edges or trimming avulsed tendons or nerves. Poorly perfused muscle should also be removed, because it will form either fibrotic tissue leading to contracture or necrotic tissue leading to infection. Additionally, large segments of devitalized muscle tissue can lead to systemic illnesses, such as hyperkalemia or renal failure from rhabdomyolysis. The 4 Cs—color, consistency, contractility, and capacity to bleed—aid in assessing muscle. Bone fragments that lack soft tissue attachment should be considered devitalized and removed—even if such debridement results in a gap. Sufficient débridement of devitalized tissues is essential in the management of the mangled hand; given its critical importance, it should most often be performed by the most senior member of the surgical team.

After débridement, the surgeon should systematically identify all damaged structures and decide whether or not limb salvage will result in a functional and sensate limb; the decision to salvage a digit or limb can be difficult. In general, the authors usually perform salvage if the operation has the possibility of resulting in useful function, but there are times that amputation of a limb (or part) is the most prudent decision. Mangled injuries may result in a stiff, painful, insensate, or functionless limb, which may require extensive therapy and multiple operations if salvage is undertaken. Although each case is different and should be considered individually, relative indications for amputation (instead of salvage) include a mangled single/border digit, segmental injury, excessive contamination, severe articular destruction, medical instability or comorbidities, perceived lack of compliance with postoperative requirements, self-inflicted injury, and/or prolonged ischemia time.[7]

The art of reconstruction of the mangled hand comes from experience in dealing with these difficult injuries. Surgeons must apply a variety of concepts to create the best extremity possible.

Order of Repair

The nature of injured structures often dictates the order of repair. If an injury is proximal and the distal part (including the intrinsic muscles of the hand) is dysvascular, a vascular shunt may be useful to establish reperfusion and prevent ischemic injury. The authors typically use a 1-mm to 3-mm shunt depending on the caliber of the vessel to be cannulated. Prior to reperfusion, there should be awareness of the possibility of metabolic sequelae of reperfusion, for which the anesthesia team should be prepared. The shunt remains in place until the vascular anastomosis is ready to be performed.

Many mangled injuries to the hand are multidigit injuries, and consideration should first be given to either the part-by-part or digit-by-digit approach. In the part-by-part approach, a surgeon repairs the same anatomic structure of each digit sequentially (first bones and then tendons, vessels, nerves, and so forth). Advantages to this approach include speed and rhythm. Alternatively, in the digit-by-digit approach, the surgeon repairs all structures in each digit sequentially. This may decrease the ischemic time for the prioritized digits. In general, the authors typically use the part-by-part approach with injuries in which the intent is to salvage all digits (because this is most expeditious) and the digit-by-digit approach for injuries in which there are unsalvageable parts and priority must be given to the most important digits for reconstruction.

If the ischemia time allows, a common order of fixation includes bone, extensor tendon, flexor tendon, artery, nerve, vein, and skin. Often, however, the authors' preference is the veins before arteries approach, in which the order of fixation includes bones, extensor tendons, veins, flexor tendons, arteries, nerves, and skin. Performing the venous anastomosis first allows this to be performed under tourniquet control and allows the surgeon to perform the most technically demanding part of the procedure prior to the onset of inevitable technical fatigue at the end of the operation. Additionally, repairing the artery first creates bleeding from the veins, which clouds the operative field and makes an already difficult step more difficult. The order of approach depends on surgeon preference and specifics of the injury.

Spare Parts and Heterotopic Replantation

When planning a reconstruction, surgeons should always consider using the parts of a nonreplantable structure. For example, a nonreconstructible index finger amputation may provide nerve, skin, bone, tendon, or arterial grafts to an adjacent digit. Additionally, priority to replanting the most intact digits should be given to the least damaged amputated fingers (eg, if an amputated index finger is better preserved than an amputated thumb, then the index finger may be replanted to the thumb position to optimize overall function). That is, it is important to use the best remaining structures to create the most functional resultant hand (**Fig. 2**).

Debate exists on the importance of each digit. The thumb contributes approximately 40% of hand function and thus is often given the first priority for reconstruction.[8,9] The radial-sided digits restore precision pinch and chuck pinch, whereas the ulnar-sided digits restore the width of the hand and power grasp.[10] Thus, given the situation, a surgeon may decide to use certain parts of the injured hand. Soucacos and colleagues[11] described 5 indications in which heterotopic replantation is indicated (**Box 2**).[11] The authors' preference is to reconstruct the thumb first followed by the long and ring fingers to provide opposition, pinch, and grasp.

Ectopic replantation is another option for highly damaged limbs in which radical débridement would lead to loss of important structures. Examples include burns, gunshot wounds, segmental trauma, and agricultural inquiries. The first report of ectopic replantation was published by Godina and colleagues,[12] who replanted a hand to the thoracodorsal artery. The hand was transferred to the limb 66 days later after multiple débridements.[12] Other options for ectopic replantation include the groin, axilla, and proximal arm.[13,14]

Skeletal Fixation

Most mangled hand injuries are stabilized by external or internal fixation. In general, the authors prefer internal fixation when possible, because it allows for earlier mobilization and can provide long-term fixation. External fixation can be useful and expeditious in severe injuries and those with gross instability or contamination; placing

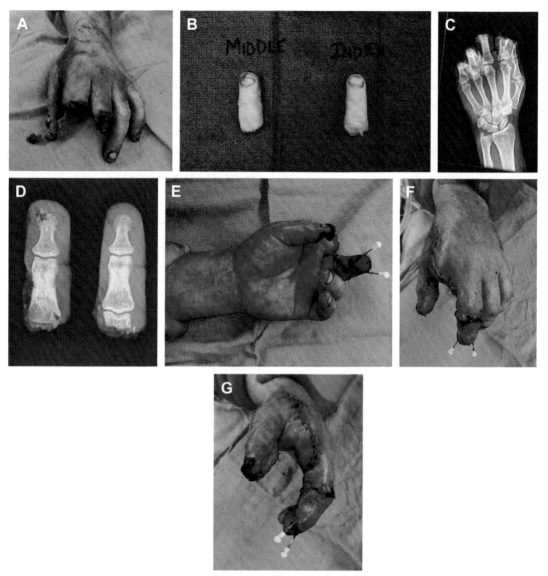

Fig. 2. Spare parts can be useful. This patient sustained amputations of the index and middle fingers and a de-gloving soft tissue injury to the volar aspect of his left thumb (*A*). The index finger amputation level was 1 cm proximal to the proximal interphalangeal joint, and the middle finger amputation level was directly through the proximal interphalangeal joint (*B-D*). The patient underwent heterotopic replantation of the amputated index finger (IF) to the middle finger (MF) position (*E*). He subsequently underwent ray amputation of the index finger with first dorsal metacarpal artery flap reconstruction of the volar thumb defect (*F,G*).

permanent hardware in highly contaminated wounds raises the risk for infection, and medically unstable patients may not tolerate the second trauma of a long operation (damage control surgery).[15]

In the wrist, the authors often use plate fixation with or without percutaneous Kirschner wires; a radial-carpal internal spanning plate (ie, for wrist fusion) can be useful in cases of significant bony injury to the wrist. For the digits, the authors prefer small plates or 90/90 wiring constructs, which provide adequate stabilization. Additionally, the authors usually shorten the bone prior to fixation to relax the tension on the microsurgical vessel and nerve repairs.

If significant bone loss is present, a choice may be to acutely bone graft the defect, possibly from spare parts. Unlike the lower extremity, acute bone grafting in the upper extremity does not seem to have the same risk for infection.[16] Alternatively, if the wound is contaminated, the space may be filled with antibiotic impregnated beads

Box 2
Indications for heterotopic replantation

1. In a multifinger injury where the thumb is not replantable, the best-preserved digit is transferred to the thumb position.

2. In a bilateral thumb amputation, the dominant thumb is given the best-preserved thumb or digit.

3. In bilateral multidigit amputations, the dominant hand is given the best-preserved digits.

4. In multidigit amputations with an intact thumb, the ulnar-sided positions are given the best-preserved digits to restore grasp.

5. In amputations including all 5 digits, the best-preserved parts are given to restore the thumb first, followed by the ulnar digits.

or a cement spacer, which can later be replaced with cancellous autograft (Masquelet procedure) or structural cortical graft (such as iliac crest).[17] Large segments of bone loss (greater than 6 cm) may benefit from vascularized bone transport or free vascularized bone flaps.[18]

Tendon Repair

Most tendon lacerations can be repaired using standard techniques involving core-locking sutures with an epitendinous running stitch. The authors prefer to run the epitendinous stitch first to avoid bunching and facilitate speed.[19] Most importantly, tendon edges should be débrided of nonviable tissue. Segmental gaps can occasionally be treated with autograft from palmaris longus or from an amputated spare part. If tendon transfers are considered, the authors often perform these in staged fashion after tissue equilibrium has occurred. Large segmental tendon defects or defects in the flexor tendon sheath can be treated in a staged fashion. A silicone Hunter rod can be placed in either the flexor or extensor side to create a sheath for future reconstruction.

Vascular Repair

In the setting of vascular injury, vessel repair is critical to the survival and function of the limb and includes both arterial and venous repair. The technical details of microsurgical anastomoses are beyond the scope of this article, but it is critical for surgeons to adequately prepare and débride the vessels and position themselves optimally for technical success. For dysvascular digits, the authors typically recommend repairing a minimum of 2 digital veins for each artery repaired, which has been correlated with increased survival.[20]

Another important consideration with mangled hand reconstruction is the potential need for a vein graft. Injuries with a crush or avulsion component often require a vein graft because of the extent of vascular injury. The vessel diameter should match the artery, and it is often taken from the volar wrist or the foot/ankle. Larger vessels of the forearm may require harvesting the greater or lesser saphenous vein. For injuries involving the arch, vein grafts with a reversed Y configuration can be harvested, often from the dorsal foot, to reconstruct the common digital arterial branches.

Microsurgical repair can fail for numerous reasons. (1) If the repair is performed on an injured vessel, the surgeon must evaluate the vessel under the operating microscope and débride proximal and distal vessel ends to an uninjured segment. Parts that appear kinked (ribbon sign) or bruised (red line sign) should be resected. Adequate débridement is confirmed by observing robust, pulsatile blood flow from the proximal segment. (2) Failure can also occur from technical error, which should be immediately recognized and remedied. (3) Microvascular failure can also occur from infection, which causes vasoconstriction and thrombosis. (4) Failure can occur from excessive extrinsic compression. To avoid compression, the authors perform fasciotomies for proximal injuries, a loose skin closure to allow egress of blood or serous fluid, liberal use of skin grafts, and loose dressings with nothing in between the fingers. (5) Failure can occur from inadequate venous outflow; congestion causes a reduction in inflow followed by necrosis.

Nerve Repair

A perfused limb or digit without sensation is not functional. Nerve repair in the setting of a mangled limb is often performed near the end of the procedure but often is one of the more important parts of surgery. Lacerated or avulsed nerves should be débrided back to healthy fascicles under the microscope. This can be confirmed by palpation of the nerve ends, visualization of pooching fascicles, and the presence of endoneurial bleeding. A tensionless repair should be achieved, or alternative methods of neurrorhaphy should be used (ie, conduit, allograft, or autograft repair). When a nerve gap is present, a small gap (<10 mm) can be bridged with a nerve conduit[21] whereas larger nerve gaps should often be bridged with allograft or autograft.[22] Generally speaking, it is the authors' practice to perform nerve repair or reconstruction at the time of the initial surgery regardless of the method required.

Soft Tissue Coverage

Soft tissue coverage should be considered at the time of initial evaluation, because this is an important aspect of recovery and paramount to allow for gliding of critical structures. Most often, primary closure is possible and is the first choice. It is important to close the skin loosely to allow for drainage and egress of fluid.

If primary closure is not possible, healing by secondary intention is another option and may be appropriate in small defects. Other times, skin grafting may be sufficient for coverage but generally is inadequate over bone devoid of periosteum or tendon without paratenon.

For larger defects, temporary coverage with Integra or a negative pressure wound device may be the best option for initial management. In the authors' experience, larger defects commonly require flap coverage and the preference is to perform this within 1 week postinjury, assuming the wound is sufficiently clean and adequately débrided. Early soft tissue coverage for mutilating injuries has been shown in studies to decrease late infection.[23] A variety of local, regional, and free flaps exist for this purpose (**Table 1**). Definitive flap coverage may occur acutely or as part of staged protocol when a wound is clean and fully débrided. In the current era of routine microsurgery, it is the authors' opinion that free flap

Table 1
Common flaps for upper extremity reconstruction

Flap	Dominant Vessel	Destination
V-Y advancement	Random	Transverse or dorsal oblique finger tip
Rotational	Random	Dorsal hand or forearm
Cross-finger	Random	Volar finger
Thenar	Random	Finger tip
Moberg	Thumb digital arteries	Volar tip of thumb
First dorsal metacarpal artery	First dorsal metacarpal artery	Dorsal or volar thumb
Posterior interosseous artery	Posterior interosseous artery	Dorsal hand or forearm
Reverse radial forearm	Radial artery	Volar hand, web space, dorsal hand
Reverse lateral arm	Posterior radial collateral artery	Elbow or free flap to cover hand or forearm
Groin	Superficial circumflex iliac artery	Hand or forearm
Abdominal	Medial or lateral row perforators of deep inferior epigastric artery	Hand or forearm
Anterolateral thigh	Descending branch of lateral femoral circumflex artery	Free flap to cover hand or forearm
Gracilis	Branches of medial femoral circumflex	Free-functioning muscle transfer with neurorrhaphy to obturator nerve for forearm or arm
Latissimus dorsi	Thoracodorsal artery	Pedicled or free flap to cover the upper extremity
Fibula	Peroneal artery	Free osseous flap for bony defects in the arm or forearm
Medial femoral condyle	Descending genicular artery	Free flap for osseous defects in the forearm or hand
Great toe	First dorsal metatarsal artery (from dorsalis pedis) or plantar digital artery (from lateral plantar artery)	Free flap for thumb or finger reconstruction with digital nerve and tendons

coverage is, at times, the safest and most expeditious way to cover difficult wounds, and sacrificing the anterograde radial (or ulnar) arterial inflow is rarely chosen.

POSTOPERATIVE MANAGEMENT

The limb should be placed in a loose dressing, usually involving a plaster splint, and elevated. Patients with heavily contaminated wounds may require repeat débridement within 24 hours to 48 hours. It is imperative to débride all nonviable tissue prior to definitive coverage.

For those patients undergoing revascularization, the authors use a warm environment (warm room, heating device such as a warming blanket, or both) and daily aspirin. Most often, the authors do not use adjunctive anticoagulants, such as heparin, enoxaparin, or dextran, unless there is a clinical reason to do so. Monitoring for perfusion usually occurs every hour for the first 24 hours postoperatively, which consists of continuous pulse oximetry on 1 or more of the digits and evaluation of skin color, turgor, capillary refill, temperature, and Doppler pulse. Arterial insufficiency is heralded by pallor, flaccid turgor, slow refill, cool temperature, reduced oximetry, and absent pulse. Venous insufficiency is heralded by violaceous color, engorged tissues, brisk capillary refill, low temperature, and low or normal oximetry reading, often with a present pulse. Some of these features can be difficult to distinguish in individuals with darker skin (**Fig. 3**), and it is critical to have experienced nursing for care of these patients.

Arterial insufficiency requires immediate exploration if an attempt at salvage is to be made; the surgeon is required to evaluate the anastomosis and repair or vein graft the segment if thrombosis is present. Venous insufficiency can, at times, be treated with controlled bleeding with either leech therapy or rubbing the nail bed periodically with a heparin-soaked pledget. If leeches are used,

antibiotic prophylaxis with ciprofloxacin is added to cover *Aeromonas hydrophila*. In general, the authors return to the operating room immediately for vascular issues after proximal extremity injuries and thumb revascularization but are more selective with single digits, particularly if there are multiple injured components.

Intravenous antibiotics are continued for 48 hours to 72 hours after the last débridement. In general, the authors usually begin some form of passive motion therapy and splinting before discharge; however, this is dependent on the injury and the restrictions on tendon gliding and early motion. Patients usually remain on an aspirin for 1 month. The first postoperative visit occurs within a week of discharge and focuses on wound care, soft tissue viability, and motion. At this visit, it is important for patients to understand the nature of their injuries and the expectations and requirements for recovery.

In patients with mangled upper extremity injuries, secondary procedures are often necessary. Tenolysis and capsulotomy are the most common secondary procedures usually occurring in the first 3 months to 6 months. Other considerations include reconstructive options for additional soft tissue coverage, bone loss or nonunion, tendon transfers, nerve grafting or transfers, toe transfers, and vascularized composite allotransplantation.[24] Secondary procedures are tailored to a patient's functional needs and wishes for additional intervention.

OUTCOMES

Outcomes are difficult to assess due to the vast heterogeneity of injuries. Scoring systems have emerged based on pain, motion, sensation, ability to work and care for oneself, and patient satisfaction.[25,26] For replanted digits, survival rates are reported between 57% and 92%.[26–36] Favorable factors for survival include well-preserved part,

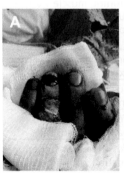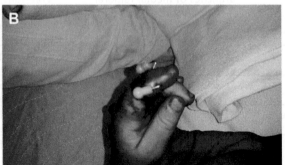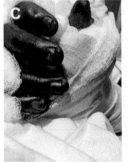

Fig. 3. Examples of vascular insufficiencies. (*A*) Arterial insufficiency. (*B*) Venous insufficiency. (*C*) Insufficiency highlighting the difficulty in dark-pigmented individuals.

sharp injury, radial-sided digit, no history of tobacco use, and no concurrent life-saving surgery.

With appropriate salvage, outcomes can be good. Finger replantation was shown in a review by Hattori and colleagues[30] to have superior appearance and function compared with amputation. Graham and colleagues[31] reviewed amputations proximal to the wrist and found superior functional scores with replantation compared with revision amputation/prosthetic fitting. Function seems to correlate with the mechanism of injury, the level of injury, severity of injury, and ischemic time. Range of motion is usually greater in amputation levels outside of flexor tendon zone 2. Paavilainen and colleagues[32] reported on transmetacarpal replantations that measured a final average total arc of motion of 154° with the mean grip and pinch strength measured at 56% and 58% of the unaffected side, respectively. Sears and Chung[33] reported an average total arc of motion of 174° in finger avulsion injuries. The functional outcomes of proximal limb replantation are significantly inferior compared with distal injuries. Hierner and colleagues[34] reported that a "functional" upper extremity could be reconstructed in 25% of upper arm replantations, 30% of proximal forearm replantations, and 58% of distal forearm replantations. Recovery of sensibility is more favorable for younger patients, sharp injuries, and distal injuries; in a series of 400 digital replantations, Glickman and Mackinnon[35] noted an average 2-point discrimination of 8 mm in sharp amputations and 15 mm in crush avulsion injuries.[35]

In conclusion, although a variety of factors may alter the outcome, reasonable expectations of limb salvage include approximately 75% to 80% survival, half the strength and motion of the unaffected side, and recovery of protective sensation in most distal injuries. If done well, patients can achieve superior function and are grateful with upper extremity limb salvage. Patients should understand that longer recovery, risk, cost, and multiple procedures, however, are usually required to achieve that goal.

REFERENCES

1. Pederson WC. Replantation. Plast Reconstr Surg 2001;107:823–41.
2. Chung KC, Spilson SV. The frequency and epidemiology of hand and forearm fractures in the United States. J Hand Surg 2001;26(5):908–15.
3. Wilhelmi BJ, Lee WPA, Pagenstert GI, et al. Replantation in the mutilated hand. Hand Clin 2003;19(1): 89–120.
4. Wei FC, Chang YL, Chen HC, et al. Three successful digital replantations in a patient after 84, 86, and 94 hours of cold ischemia time. Plast Reconstr Surg 1988;82(2):346–50.
5. VanderWilde RS, Wood MB, Zu ZG. Hand replantation after 54 hours of cold ischemia: a case report. J Hand Surg Am 1992;17(2):217–20.
6. Tarabadkar N, Iorio ML, Gundle K, et al. The use of pulse oximetry for objective quantification of vascular injuries in the hand. Plast Reconstr Surg 2015;136(6):1227–33.
7. Soucacos PN. Indications and selection for digital amputation and replantation. J Hand Surg 2001; 26B:572–81.
8. Chow JA, Bilos ZJ, Chunprapaph B. Thirty thumb replantations. Indications and results. Plast Reconstr Surg 1979;64(5):626–30.
9. Earley MJ, Watson JS. Twenty four thumb replantations. J Hand Surg Br 1984;9(1):98–102.
10. Rose EH, Buncke HJ. Selective finger transposition and primary metacarpal ray resection in multidigit amputations of the hand. J Hand Surg Am 1983; 8(2):178–82.
11. Soucacos PN, Beris AE, Malizos KN, et al. Transpositional microsurgery in multiple digital amputations. Microsurgery 1994;15(7):469–73.
12. Godina M, Bajec J, Baraga A. Salvage of the mutilated upper extremity with temporary ectopic implantation of the undamaged part. Plast Reconstr Surg 1986;78(3):295–9.
13. Higgins J. Ectopic banking of amputated parts: a clinical review. J Hand Surg Am 2011;36(11): 1868–76.
14. Valerio IL, Hui-Chou HG, Zelken J, et al. Ectopic banking of amputated great toe for delayed thumb reconstruction: case report. J Hand Surg Am 2014; 39(7):1323–6.
15. Pape HC, Giannoudis P, Krettek C. The timing of fracture treatment in polytrauma patients: relevance of damage control orthopedic surgery. Am J Surg 2002;183(6):622–9.
16. Saint-Cyr M, Gupta A. Primary internal fixation and bone grafting for open fractures of the hand. Hand Clin 2006;22(3):317–27.
17. Micev AJ, Kalainov DM, Soneru AP. Masquelet technique for treatment of segmental bone loss in the upper extremity. J Hand Surg Am 2015;40(3):593–8.
18. Wei FC, Chen HC, Chuang CC, et al. Fibular osteoseptocutaneous flap: anatomic study and clinical application. Plast Reconstr Surg 1986;78:191–9.
19. Chang J, Jones N. Twelve simple maneuvers to optimize digital replantation and revascularization. Tech Hand Up Extrem Surg 2004;8(3):161–6.
20. Efanov JI, Rizis D, Landes G, et al. Impact of the number of veins repaired in short-term digital replantation survival rate. J Plast Reconstr Aesthet Surg 2016;69(5):640–5.

21. Safa B, Buncke G. Autograft substitutes: conduits and processed nerve allografts. Hand Clin 2016; 32(2):127–40.

22. Cho MS, Rinker BD, Weber RV, et al. Functional outcome following nerve repair in the upper extremity using processed nerve allograft. J Hand Surg Am 2012;37(11):2340–9.

23. Godina M. Early microsurgical reconstruction of complex trauma of the extremities. Plast Reconstr Surg 1986;78(3):285–92.

24. Yu JC, Shieh SJ, Lee JW, et al. Secondary procedures following digital replantation and revascularisation. Br J Plast Surg 2003;56(2):125–8.

25. Chen ZW, Yu HL. Current procedures in China on replantation of severed limbs and digits. Clin Orthop 1987;215:15–23.

26. Tamai S. Twenty years' experience of limb replantation—review of 293 upper extremity replants. J Hand Surg 1982;7:549–56.

27. Fufa D, Calfee R, Wall L, et al. Digit replantation: experience of two U.S. academic level-I trauma centers. J Bone Joint Surg Am 2013;95:2127–34.

28. Waikakul S, Sakkarnkosol S, Vanadurongwan V, et al. Results of 1018 digital replantations in 552 patients. Injury 2000;31:33–40.

29. Waikakul S, Vanadurongwan V, Unnanuntana A. Prognostic factors for major limb re-implantation at both immediate and long-term follow-up. J Bone Joint Surg Br 1998;80:1024–30.

30. Hattori Y, Doi K, Ikeda K, et al. A retrospective study of functional outcomes after successful replantation versus amputation closure for single fingertip amputations. J Hand Surg 2006;31A:811–8.

31. Graham B, Adkins P, Tsai TM, et al. Major replantation versus revision amputation and prosthetic fitting in the upper extremity: a late functional outcomes study. J Hand Surg 1998;23A:783–91.

32. Paavilainen P, Nietosvaara Y, Tikkinen KA, et al. Long-term results of transmetacarpal replantation. J Plast Reconstr Aesthet Surg 2007;60:704–9.

33. Sears ED, Chung KC. Replantation of finger avulsion injuries: a systematic review of survival and functional outcomes. J Hand Surg Am 2011;36: 686–94.

34. Hierner R, Berger A, Brenner P. Considerations on the management of subtotal and total macro-amputation of the upper extremity. Unfallchirurg 1998;101(3):184–92 [in German].

35. Glickman LT, Mackinnon SE. Sensory recovery following digital replantation. Microsurgery 1990; 11:236–42.

36. Wei FC, Chuang CC, Chen HC, et al. Ten-digit replantation. Plast Reconstr Surg 1984;74(6): 826–32.

Carpal Tunnel Syndrome and Distal Radius Fractures

David Pope, MD[a], Peter Tang, MD, MPH, FAOA[b],*

KEYWORDS

- Acute carpal tunnel syndrome • Distal radius fractures • Nerve compression • Carpal tunnel release

KEY POINTS

- Three types of carpal tunnel syndrome occur after a distal radius fracture: acute, subacute or transient, and delayed.
- Acute carpal tunnel syndrome is likely caused by increases in carpal tunnel pressure and presents with progressive pain and median nerve dysfunction immediately after a distal radius fracture.
- Acute carpal tunnel syndrome should be treated with expeditious carpal tunnel release and fracture fixation.
- Subacute or transient carpal tunnel syndrome can frequently be treated with observation alone initially.
- Delayed carpal tunnel syndrome is typically due to alterations in carpal tunnel anatomy and requires etiology-specific treatment.

INTRODUCTION

Distal radius fractures (DRFs) are the most common fracture seen in the emergency department, with an incidence greater than 640,000 fractures per year.[1] Complications of DRF are many and include malunion, arthrosis, nonunion, tendon ruptures, complex regional pain syndrome, loss of motion at the wrist or fingers, compartment syndrome, and carpal tunnel syndrome (CTS).[2,3] It was not until 1933, when Abbott and Saunders[4] published a review of 9 cases, that the association of DRF and CTS was recognized as a more common phenomenon. CTS after DRF can be divided into 3 categories: acute, transient, and delayed.

Acute CTS, with an incidence of 5.4% to 8.6% after a DRF, is characterized by progressive pain and paresthesias in the median nerve distribution of the hand that develops over hours to days after a fracture. Its etiology is presumed likely due to elevated compartment pressure in the carpal tunnel.[3,5–8] In contrast, transient CTS, with an estimated incidence of 4%, has the least understood etiology of the 3 but is likely due to nerve contusion and/or stretch.[9] Unlike acute CTS, the symptoms of transient CTS can be present at the time of injury but classically do not progress, but rather gradually improve over days to weeks.[4,9,10] Lastly, delayed CTS, with an incidence of 0.5% to 22% after a DRF, can present months to years after an injury and is usually due to an alteration of the

Disclosure Statement: Speaker's Bureau: AxoGen, Inc. Depuy Synthes. Consultant: Globus Medical. Previous research funding from the Orthopaedic Research and Education Foundation (OREF), Orthopaedic Scientific Research Foundation (OSRF), American Association for Hand Surgery (AAHS), American Foundation for Surgery of the Hand (AFSH), and AxoGen, Inc (P. Tang). D. Pope – No disclosures.

[a] Department of Orthopaedic Surgery, Allegheny General Hospital, 1307 Federal Street, Federal North Building, 2nd Floor, Pittsburgh, PA 15212, USA; [b] Department of Orthopaedic Surgery, Allegheny General Hospital, Drexel University College of Medicine, 1307 Federal Street, Federal North Building, 2nd Floor, Pittsburgh, PA 15212, USA
* Corresponding author.
E-mail address: peter.tang@ahn.org

Hand Clin 34 (2018) 27–32
https://doi.org/10.1016/j.hcl.2017.09.003
0749-0712/18/© 2017 Elsevier Inc. All rights reserved.

carpal tunnel anatomy after healing of the fracture.[3,8,11–14]

ACUTE CARPAL TUNNEL SYNDROME
Pathophysiology

Acute CTS after DRF is believed to be caused by a rapid increase in carpal tunnel pressure.[8,15,16] Increased carpal tunnel pressure can be due to traumatic wrist deformity with fracture displacement, hematoma formation, displaced volar fragments, generalized edema, local anesthetic injection, and wrist immobilization in excessive flexion or extension.[15–18] Gelberman and colleagues[16] evaluated carpal tunnel pressures in patients with DRFs and found that 45% of fractured wrists placed in 40° of flexion had carpal canal pressures greater than 40 mm Hg. Other factors that predispose patients to acute CTS include high-energy injuries, ipsilateral upper extremity trauma, women under the age of 48, multiple closed reduction attempts, DRF with greater than 35% fracture translation, fractures with significant comminution (AO type C), and radiocarpal dislocations.[6,7,18]

Diagnosis

It is essential that diagnosis of acute CTS after DRF be made in an expeditious fashion because a delay or missed diagnosis can lead to nerve injury and/or nerve dysfunction, such as complex regional pain syndrome.[19–21] Unrelenting pain and dysesthesias in the median nerve distribution of the hand are the hallmark symptoms of acute CTS. The sensory examination likely reveals altered 2-point discrimination and Semmes-Weinstein monofilament testing (monofilament testing being the most sensitive way to detect sensory threshold changes) in the median nerve distribution.[20] Other examination findings can include thenar motor weakness and a positive stretch test (pain at the volar wrist with passive extension of the fingers).[22]

Beyond examination findings, a diagnosis of acute CTS can also be made by measuring carpal tunnel compartment pressure. This can be done by inserting a wick catheter or the needle of an Stryker brand Intra-Compartmental (STIC) Pressure Monitor STIC device (Stryker, Kalamazoo, Michigan) 1 cm proximal to the wrist crease and just ulnar to the palmaris longus or in line with the ring finger ray if the palmaris longus is absent. The catheter is directed 45° distally and dorsally in a slightly radial direction until it sits just radial to the hook of the hamate[23] (**Fig. 1**). Mack and colleagues[23] suggest checking carpal tunnel pressure if the symptoms do not resolve within 2 hours of elevation

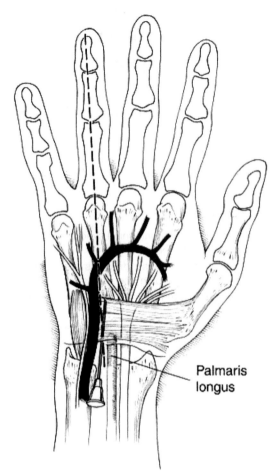

Palmaris longus

Fig. 1. Recommended catheter placement in the ulnar aspect of the carpal tunnel. (*From* Schnetzler KA. Acute carpal tunnel syndrome. J Am Acad Orthop Surg 2008;16[5]:280; with permission.)

and cast/dressing release. A pressure of greater than 30 mm Hg in the carpal tunnel can be considered diagnostic for acute CTS.

Treatment

The treatment of acute CTS is immediate carpal tunnel release (CTR) with provisional or definitive fracture reduction and/or stabilization. In particular, any gross bony deformity or displaced bony fragments that impinge on the median nerve are corrected. Most investigators recommend immediate release of the carpal tunnel to achieve best outcomes.[3,14,24,25] Regardless of the method of fixation of the distal radius, the carpal tunnel can be released in the standard fashion, open or mini-open. Endoscopic CTR is not recommended in this setting due to the trauma and altered anatomy. If volar locked plating with a volar approach is planned for fracture fixation, it is preferable to use a separate dedicated incision for the CTR to avoid inadvertent injury to the palmar cutaneous branch of the median nerve by connecting the 2 incisions.[26] Alternative techniques includes a hybrid flexor carpi radialis (FCR) approach.[26] Although there is no clear superior surgical technique for how best to release the carpal tunnel, it is clear that patients without signs of preoperative median nerve dysfunction after a DRF should not undergo a prophylactic CTR.[27,28]

For acute CTS, the preference of the senior author (P.T.) is to perform a standard open CTR, which is larger than a standard miniopen incision (miniopen incision measures 1.7–2.0 cm and starts 5 mm distal to the wrist flexion crease). The standard open CTR starts at the wrist flexion crease and is used to allow better inspection of the nerve within the carpal tunnel after the release (**Fig. 2**). A separate incision for the fracture approach and fixation is then longitudinally centered over the FCR tendon up to but not crossing the distal wrist flexion crease.

TRANSIENT CARPAL TUNNEL SYNDROME

Transient, or subacute, CTS after DRF is characterized by transient median nerve dysfunction that starts immediately after the injury and does not progress. In general, this type of CTS is most frequently caused by a median nerve stretch or contusion from initial fracture displacement or volarly displaced fragments but can also be related to edema or hematoma.[4,10] On examination these patients usually do not have any objective nerve deficits but they report subjective numbness in the median nerve distribution. In these patients, median nerve dysfunction generally resolve with observation, elevation, and adequate fracture reduction.[29] Although a majority of these patients' symptoms resolve with observation alone, in patients with volarly displaced fragments some investigators recommend early CTR with removal or reduction of displaced fragments to avoid continued median nerve compression.[10,30]

The senior author's preference is to perform a CTR during fracture repair for any patient with transient CTS who have any subjective numbness in the median nerve distribution. The senior author also performs a CTR in any patient with any preinjury symptoms of CTS. The reasoning for this approach is to address a potential secondary site of compression for the median nerve (carpal tunnel) if the nerve has been injured at the level of the distal radius, which is akin to a double crush phenomenon, and also to address suspected idiopathic CTS. Furthermore, the patient is already undergoing surgery and the concomitant CTR could obviate a second surgery. In terms of surgical technique, the senior author uses a standard miniopen CTR incision

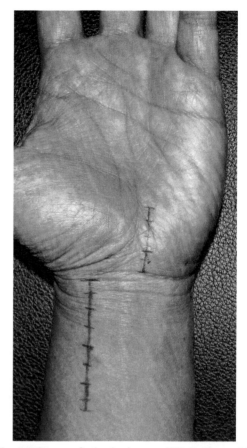

Fig. 2. Picture of standard open CTR incision with volar Henry incision. A dot is placed at the center of the distal pole of the scaphoid and well as the center of the pisiform. A dot is made at the midpoint between these first 2 marks. A dot is also placed at the wrist flexion crease in line with the radial border of the ring finger. The CTR incision is centered between the scaphoid/pisiform midpoint mark and the radial border of the ring finger mark, or the more ulnar of the 2 points. A more ulnar-based incision is preferred to avoid injury to a transligamentous motor branch with the assumption that if a transligamentous branch is present it will traverse the ligament more radially. The CTR incision starts at the wrist flexion crease and is approximately 3 cm long.

through a separate incision at the standard location at the base of the volar hand (**Fig. 3**).

DELAYED CARPAL TUNNEL SYNDROME

Delayed CTS, with an incidence of 0.5% to 22% after DRF, can present months to years after injury and is usually associated with the late effects of the altered anatomy in the carpal tunnel and not necessarily a critical increase in canal pressure. The etiology includes malunion, chronic tenosynovitis, volarly displaced fragments, cicatrix,

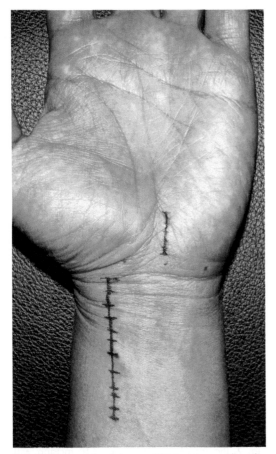

Fig. 3. Picture of miniopen CTR incision with volar Henry incision. The same landmarks are made as in **Fig. 1**. The miniopen CTR incision begins 5 mm to 8 mm distal to the wrist flexion crease and measure 1.7 cm to 2.0 cm in length.

enlarged volar callus, and prominent hardware.[3,11,12,14] The symptoms of delayed CTS after DRF are not well described in the literature but are generally assumed to be similar in presentation to idiopathic CTS.

The diagnosis of delayed CTS after a DRF follows the normal work-up for CTS once anatomic and radiographic abnormalities are assessed first. It is also possible that some patients with presumed delayed CTS may only have developed idiopathic CTS that is unrelated to their previous DRF, which would be supported if no anatomic abnormality related to the DRF is identified after radiographic evaluation of the wrist.[31]

Treatment of delayed CTS depends on the underlying cause but does not represent the emergency that is acute CTS. Moreover, up to 66% of cases of delayed CTS can avoid surgery with conservative measures (observation, splinting, and injections).[32] It is unclear, however, in the literature whether nerve conduction studies/

electromyography should guide treatment in a similar manner as it does in idiopathic CTS. In other words, should conservative treatment be reserved for those with electrodiagnostically confirmed mild compression whereas surgery should be recommended only for moderate or severe compression? Also, should surgical treatment only consist of standard release of the transverse carpal ligament, or should surgery also address any correctable issues, such as flexor tenosynovitis, prominent volar callus, prominent hardware, or residual fracture malunion? Regardless, most commonly the issue is a thickened transverse carpal tunnel ligament and/or median nerve scarring. To address these most common etiologies, a standard CTR can resolve the thickened transverse carpal tunnel ligament and a median nerve neurolysis can free the nerve from any scarring at the level of the volar plate, assuming a locked volar plate was used previously. In a small study, Ho and colleagues[32] found

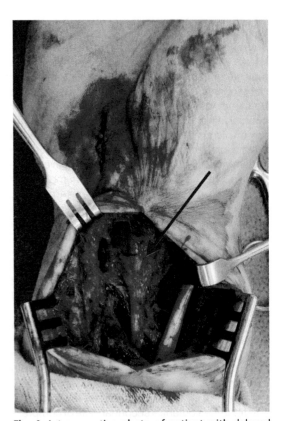

Fig. 4. Intraoperative photo of patient with delayed CTS after DRF. The initial treatment was reduction and repair of the distal radius with a locked volar plate without CTR (the patient had no median nerve symptoms at index surgery). The patient underwent a miniopen CTR and median nerve neurolysis at the distal radius level. Cicatrix formation was found encasing median nerve (*arrow*). The FCR tendon is on the right being retracted.

patients improved whether they underwent CTR alone or whether they underwent median nerve neurolysis alone. Arora and colleagues[33] noted improvement in patients with CTR and removal of hardware.

It seems that the most common cause would be cicatrix at the median nerve at the previous volar fracture repair site, so neurolysis of the nerve at the distal forearm should relieve this problem (**Fig. 4**). If this theory is correct, CTR should be unnecessary unless the carpal tunnel was released at the index procedure and this is now a site of cicatrix. If CTR was not performed at the index procedure and the problem area is the carpal tunnel, then the patient may have developed idiopathic CTS. Theoretically, nerve conduction studies/electromyography should be able to differentiate the problem area but due to the adjacent nature of the sites in question, the sensitivity of this study may be poor. Lastly, another possibility is the development of a double crush phenomenon where a patient's preexisting amount of carpal tunnel compression was not symptomatic until the nerve cicatrix formed at the distal radius level. Thus, for delayed CTS, to address any potential sites of median nerve compression, the senior author's preference is to perform a CTR (using an extended incision if CTR was done at the index procedure), median nerve neurolysis at the distal forearm with or without nerve conduit wrapping depending on the amount of scarring, and removal of the volar locked plate if present (**Fig. 5**). The

CTR would be performed whether or not the patient had a CTR at the index procedure.

SUMMARY

CTS after DRF can be categorized as acute, transient, and delayed. Early and expeditious treatment of acute CTS is necessary, and failing to diagnose and treat it can lead to permanent median nerve dysfunction. Many patients with transient CTS after DRF do not require surgical release of the carpal tunnel. For patients with delayed CTS, all possible causes of nerve compression (fracture fragments, hardware, synovitis, and so forth) should be considered and subsequently addressed. Prophylactic CTR in the absence of signs and symptoms of CTS after DRF is not indicated.

REFERENCES

1. Chung KC, Spilson SV. The frequency and epidemiology of hand and forearm fractures in the United States. J Hand Surg Am 2001;26(5):908–15.
2. Wolfe S. Green's operative hand surgery. 6th edition. Philadelphia: Elsevier/Churchill Livingstone; 2010.
3. Cooney WP 3rd, Dobyns JH, Linscheid RL. Complications of Colles' fractures. J Bone Joint Surg Am 1980;62(4):613–9.
4. Abbot L, Saunders J. Injuries of the median nerve in fracture of the lower end of the radius. Surg Gynecol Obstet 1933;57:507–16.
5. Adamson JE, Srouji SJ, Horton CE, et al. The acute carpal tunnel syndrome. Plast Reconstr Surg 1971; 47(4):332–6.
6. Bruske J, Niedzwiedz Z, Bednarski M, et al. Acute carpal tunnel syndrome after distal radius fractures–long term results of surgical treatment with decompression and external fixator application. Chir Narzadow Ruchu Ortop Pol 2002;67(1):47–53 [in Polish].
7. Dyer G, Lozano-Calderon S, Gannon C, et al. Predictors of acute carpal tunnel syndrome associated with fracture of the distal radius. J Hand Surg Am 2008;33(8):1309–13.
8. Niver GE, Ilyas AM. Carpal tunnel syndrome after distal radius fracture. Orthop Clin North Am 2012; 43(4):521–7.
9. Aro H, Koivunen T, Katevuo K, et al. Late compression neuropathies after Colles' fractures. Clin Orthop Relat Res 1988;233:217–25.
10. Kinley DL, Evarts CM. Carpal tunnel syndrome due to a small displaced fragment of bone. Report of a case. Cleve Clin Q 1968;35(4):215–21.
11. Lewis D, Miller EM. Peripheral nerve injuries associated with fractures. Ann Surg 1922;76(4):528–38.
12. Watson-Jones R. Leri's pleonosteosis, carpal tunnel compression of the median nerves and Morton's

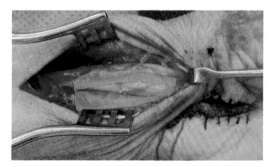

Fig. 5. Intraoperative photo of patient with delayed CTS after DRF. The initial treatment was reduction and repair of the distal radius with a locked volar plate and CTR for subacute CTS. Because this was a revision CTR setting, a longer incision was made distal and proximal to the previous incision. The proximal extent of the incision crosses the wrist flexion crease in an ulnar direction (to avoid injury to the palmar cutaneous nerve). Cicatrix was also found around the median nerve at the level of the plate. Median nerve neurolysis at the distal radius level was performed as well as removal of the volar plate. A nerve conduit (*gray shading*) was placed around the median nerve to try to prevent future scarring.

metatarsalgia. J Bone Joint Surg Br 1949;31B(4): 560–71.

13. Zachary R. Thenar palsy due to compression of the median nerve in the carpal tunnel. Surg Gynecol Obstet 1945;81:213–21.

14. Lynch AC, Lipscomb PR. The carpal tunnel syndrome and Colles' fractures. JAMA 1963;185:363–6.

15. Kongsholm J, Olerud C. Carpal tunnel pressure in the acute phase after Colles' fracture. Arch Orthop Trauma Surg 1986;105(3):183–6.

16. Gelberman RH, Garfin SR, Hergenroeder PT, et al. Compartment syndromes of the forearm: diagnosis and treatment. Clin Orthop Relat Res 1981;161: 252–61.

17. McCarroll HR Jr. Nerve injuries associated with wrist trauma. Orthop Clin North Am 1984;15(2):279–87.

18. Bauman TD, Gelberman RH, Mubarak SJ, et al. The acute carpal tunnel syndrome. Clin Orthop Relat Res 1981;156:151–6.

19. Young BT, Rayan GM. Outcome following nonoperative treatment of displaced distal radius fractures in low-demand patients older than 60 years. J Hand Surg Am 2000;25(1):19–28.

20. Nishimura A, Ogura T, Hase H, et al. Evaluation of sensory function after median nerve decompression in carpal tunnel syndrome using the current perception threshold test. J Orthop Sci 2003;8(4):500–4.

21. Puchalski P, Zyluk A. Complex regional pain syndrome type 1 after fractures of the distal radius: a prospective study of the role of psychological factors. J Hand Surg Br 2005;30(6):574–80.

22. Dresing K, Peterson T, Schmit-Neuerburg KP. Compartment pressure in the carpal tunnel in distal fractures of the radius: a prospective study. Arch Orthop Trauma Surg 1994;113:285–9.

23. Mack GR, McPherson SA, Lutz RB. Acute median neuropathy after wrist trauma. The role of emergent carpal tunnel release. Clin Orthop Relat Res 1994; 300:141–6.

24. Sponsel KH, Palm ET. Carpal tunnel syndrome following Colles' fracture. Surg Gynecol Obstet 1965;121(6):1252–6.

25. Chauhan A, Bowlin TC, Mih AD, et al. Patient-reported outcomes after acute carpal tunnel release in patients with distal radius open reduction internal fixation. Hand (N Y) 2012;7(2):147–50.

26. Gwathmey FW Jr, Brunton LM, Pensy RA, et al. Volar plate osteosynthesis of distal radius fractures with concurrent prophylactic carpal tunnel release using a hybrid flexor carpi radialis approach. J Hand Surg Am 2010;35(7):1082–8.e4.

27. Odumala O, Ayekoloye C, Packer G. Prophylactic carpal tunnel decompression during buttress plating of the distal radius: is it justified? Injury 2001;32(7): 577–9.

28. Lattmann T, Dietrich M, Meier C, et al. Comparison of 2 surgical approaches for volar locking plate osteosynthesis of the distal radius. J Hand Surg Am 2008; 33(7):1135–43.

29. Schnetzler KA. Acute carpal tunnel syndrome. J Am Acad Orthop Surg 2008;16(5):276–82.

30. Paley D, McMurtry RY. Median nerve compression by volarly displaced fragments of the distal radius. Clin Orthop Relat Res 1987;215:139–47.

31. Bienek T, Kusz D, Cielinski L. Peripheral nerve compression neuropathy after fractures of the distal radius. J Hand Surg Br 2006;31(3):256–60.

32. Ho AW, Ho ST, Koo SC, et al. Hand numbness and carpal tunnel syndrome after volar plating of distal radius fracture. Hand (N Y) 2011;6(1): 34–8.

33. Arora R, Lutz M, Hennerbichler A, et al. Complications following internal fixation of unstable distal radius fracture with a palmar locking-plate. J Orthop Trauma 2007;21(5):316–22.

Open Distal Radius Fractures
Timing and Strategies for Surgical Management

Matthew L. Iorio, MD[a],*, Carl M. Harper, MD[b],
Tamara Rozental, MD[b]

KEYWORDS

• Distal radius • Open fracture • Hand trauma

KEY POINTS

• Open distal radius fractures are rare injuries and current literature consists entirely of small patient cohorts within a wide spectrum of injury severity.
• The initial evaluation necessitates a thorough bedside irrigation, antibiotics, tetanus prophylaxis, and immobilization.
• The type and extent of contamination may be more important than simply the absolute presence of contamination or size of the soft tissue defect.
• The technique of operative fixation is dictated by the fracture pattern and the degree of soft tissue injury.
• An open fracture may carry an increased risk of nonunion that may require revision, and operative planning should include this consideration.

INTRODUCTION

Despite a reported incidence of distal radius fractures of approximately 643,000 nationally annually, the rate of open fractures of the distal radius is far less frequent at approximately 6%.[1] Although the management of open distal radius fractures has improved with better identification of comorbid factors, antibiotic administration, and guidelines for operative timing, questions remain surrounding patients with variable amounts of contamination, advanced age, or low-grade soft tissue injuries. In contrast to open fractures of the lower extremity, there are fewer comparative studies to guide treatment algorithms.

This article reviews the available data, summarizes operative indications, and provides a treatment algorithm for the management of open distal radius fractures.

INJURY CLASSIFICATION AND RISK FACTORS FOR POSTOPERATIVE INFECTION

To standardize the comparison among open fractures, grading systems have been established regarding not only the fracture classification but also the severity of the soft tissue injury. The most frequently used system of open fracture classification is the Gustilo and Anderson score, encompassing wound size and both soft tissue and bone injury patterns (**Table 1**).

Disclosure Statement: The authors have no financial interests in any of the products or techniques mentioned and have received no external support related to this study.
[a] Department of Orthopaedics, Division of Plastic Surgery, Beth Israel Deaconess Medical Center, Harvard Medical School, 330 Brookline Avenue, Stoneman 10, Boston, MA 02215, USA; [b] Department of Orthopaedics, Beth Israel Deaconess Medical Center, Harvard Medical School, 330 Brookline Avenue, Stoneman 10, Boston, MA 02215, USA
* Corresponding author.
E-mail address: mattiorio@gmail.com

Hand Clin 34 (2018) 33–40
https://doi.org/10.1016/j.hcl.2017.09.004
0749-0712/18/© 2017 Elsevier Inc. All rights reserved.

Table 1
Gustilo and Anderson classification of open fractures. Note that contamination within this scale requires a minimum score of III

Grade	
I	Wound <1 cm Simple fracture pattern with minimal comminution and minimal soft tissue damage Clean
II	Wound 1–10 cm Simple fracture pattern Mild to moderate soft tissue damage Clean
IIIA	Wound >10 cm Extensive soft tissue damage but bone remains covered High energy, comminuted, or segmental fracture pattern Contaminated
IIIB	Extensive soft tissue damage with periosteal stripping Soft tissue damage precludes skin closure over bony injury High energy, comminuted, or segmental fracture pattern Contaminated
IIIC	Any open fracture associated with an arterial injury requiring repair Contaminated

Data from Gustilo RB, Anderson JT. Prevention of infection in the treatment of one thousand and twenty-five open fractures of long bones: retrospective and prospective analyses. J Bone Joint Surg Am 1976;58:453–8.

Some investigators, however, have noted a limitation of the Gustilo classification for distal radius fractures, whereas the type of contamination may be more important than simply the absolute presence of contamination or size of the soft tissue defect.[2] In a review of 42 open distal radius fractures, Glueck and colleagues[3] determined that fractures considered contaminated with a high volume of biological material (dirt/grass), bacterial reservoirs (fecal material), or extensive foreign material (road gravel/tar) may be more predictive of postoperative infection than that of the corresponding Gustilo score. Within this group, 2 patients with fecal contamination, classified as Gustilo II and IIIB, developed severe polymicrobial postoperative infections, despite early washout and antibiotic prophylaxis. Given the limitations of the Gustilo classification in accurately predicting infection risk, the investigators suggest that the type of contamination be reported in combination with the Gustilo score to provide a better estimate of infection potential.

The Oestern and Tscherne classification was created based on the extent of soft tissue disruption and associated fracture severity (**Table 2**). This score adds a prognostic component to the total injury score and demonstrates good intraobserver reliability. In a prospective evaluation of the Osetern and Tscherne classification, patients with tibial plateau and pilon fractures were consecutively evaluated at serial time points by 15 orthopedic surgeons in various stages of training and career. The overall intraobserver agreement for all 15 evaluators was substantial at 0.81 (95% CI, 0.79–0.83), whereas the interobserver agreement was moderate at 0.65 (95% CI, 0.55–0.73).[4] To date, however, the Gustilo score remains the most widely applied classification system for open injuries of the extremities.

In a review of open fractures of the distal radius, Rozental and colleagues[5] evaluated 18 patients with open distal radius fractures and found the Gustilo score a significant predictor of infection. Although the majority of patients in the cohort sustained Gustilo type I fractures (50%), most patients requiring serial débridements sustained Gustilo III injuries. In agreement with other studies, the investigators determined that type of fixation did not correlate with risk factors for postoperative infection; however, these patients were distributed among all 3 levels of Gustilo scoring (type I 29%, type II 14%, and type III 57%).

To determine potential risk factors for ongoing infection, a retrospective study of 122 patients

Table 2
Oestern and Tscherne classification of open fractures and associated soft tissue disruption

Grade	
0	Minimal soft tissue damage Simple fracture pattern
1	Skin lacerated by bone fragment No or minimal skin contusion/damage Minimal comminution
2	Skin laceration with circumferential skin or soft-tissue contusion and moderate contamination Moderate comminution or segmental fracture pattern
3	Extensive soft tissue damage with major vessel and/or nerve injury Severely comminuted fracture with bone loss likely
4	Subtotal/near total amputation

Adapted from Tscherne H, Oestern HJ. A new classification of soft-tissue damage in open and closed fractures. Unfallheilkunde 1982;85(3):111–5; with permission of Springer Nature.

was performed and a combinatorial score called the infection risk score was created combining elements of the Gustilo classification and Tscherne classification as well as the time from initial injury (<12 h, 12–24 h, and >24 h). Predictive factors for postoperative infection included a delay in time to treatment (30.3 h ±19.5 h) for the infection group versus 21.4 hours (±12.1 h for others). Additionally, the Gustilo scoring demonstrated infection in 74.2% of type III injuries, as did types 2 and 3 Tscherne injuries of (25.8% and 48.4%, respectively). The reported infection risk score had a sensitivity of 0.84 and a specificity of 0.55. Similar to other studies previously discussed, the investigators noted that the type of fixation type did not correlate with infection risk.

TIMING OF SURGICAL INTERVENTION

The timing of surgical intervention remains a source of controversy and national debate. The 6-hour rule for débridement and stabilization of open fractures, which has served as dogma, is based on only a handful of small series published prior to the regular administration of antibiotics and with a limited statistical analysis. The 1898 study of Paul Leopold Friedrich is the most cited among these and is often credited with the 6-hour rule, where wounds in the triceps of guinea pigs were surgically created and inoculated with "mud and horse dust."[6] No antibiotics were administered and débridements were performed at 30-minute intervals. The investigators reported that although all animals débrided by 6 hours survived, those débrided after 8.5 hours died. Several other basic science studies followed supporting operative débridement within 6 hours but none established a clinical correlation in human patients. As such, clinical studies to date have not established the definitive timing for surgical débridement. Moreover, a recent systematic review of open fractures of the hand by Ketonis and colleagues,[7] with 12 articles and a total of 1669 open fractures meeting the inclusion criteria, identified that the infection rate after open hand fractures remain low, but the correlation to the development of the infection related stronger to the administration to the timing of antibiotic administration and not the timing to débridement.

Kaufman and colleagues[8] demonstrated the safety of "immediate" operative débridement and surgical intervention in 21 patients at an age of 60 years or older. Despite their description of operative timing preferences, however, the investigators describe important variations in practice regarding surgical timing to allow medical optimization prior to intervention. As such, their article

may do more to demonstrate the safety of delayed intervention, with a majority of interventions occurring beyond the 12-hour mark, than to advocate for immediate surgical débridement.

Although a prospective randomized controlled trial comparing timing of operative debridement would be useful, it is logistically difficult to perform. The authors, therefore, rely on large clinical series applying current treatment methods, such as the early administration of antibiotics, to guide the management of open fractures of the distal radius. A majority of these studies have been performed in the lower extremity, specifically the tibia, because it has the highest incidence of open fracture of the long bones. Adequate soft tissue coverage not only creates a barrier of ongoing contamination toward possible osteomyelitis but also may ensure a vascular envelope around bone that may otherwise become devitalized with periosteal stripping and endosteal disruption. In comparison to lower extremity injuries, except in instances of high energy, the relatively nonadherent soft tissue envelope may be better suited to remain viable. These studies have shown that the timing of operative débridement can be safely performed within 24 hours of injury without incurring an increased risk of infection provided antibiotics are administered on presentation (5.6%–22.6% infection rate with no difference between group débrided at <6 h and the group débrided after 6 h up to 24 h).[9,10]

Unfortunately, few studies have exclusively evaluated the timing of débridement for upper extremity fractures. Swanson and colleagues[11] evaluated 200 patients with open hand fractures. At an average follow-up of 17.5 weeks (range, 1–139 wk), the investigators reported an infection rate of 7%. Although the investigators attribute this to wound contamination and systemic comorbid illness, conclusions are difficult to draw from this retrospective case series.[11]

In studies including both upper and lower extremity injuries, no difference was detected in infection rate as it relates to the timing of surgical débridement. Srour and colleagues[12] prospectively examined 315 patients with open fractures (27 upper arm, 67 forearm, 69 femur, and 152 leg) regarding Gustilo grade, fracture location, and time to operative débridement (0–6 h, 7–12 h, 13–18 h, and 18–24 h). No statistical differences were detected in terms of time to operative débridement although this was not a primary outcome of the study. Weber and colleagues[13] published a prospective cohort of 731 open fractures in the tibia/fibula (n = 413, 52%), upper extremity (n = 285, 36%), and femur (n = 93, 12%). Infection developed in 46 fractures (6%).

Multivariate regression analysis showed that a higher incidence of infection occurred in Gustilo IIIB/IIIC fractures and in fractures of the lower extremity. No difference in infection rate was found with respect to time to débridement.

Despite their inherent limitations, these series demonstrate that it is likely the degree of soft tissue injury (for which Gustilo classification functions as a surrogate) and fracture location rather than the time to operative débridement (provided it occurs within 24 h) that is the primary determinant of postoperative infection. Furthermore, evidence has demonstrated that open fractures of the upper extremity may not carry the same risk of infection as fractures of similar grade in the lower extremity.

SERIAL DÉBRIDEMENT

To date, no objective clinical guidelines exist to determine when a wound is amenable to closure. The decision to proceed with multiple débridements verses primary closure is at the discretion and experience of the operative surgeon. A balance exists between preventing nosocomial infections with immediate closure and preventing infection from primary contamination. Early work, such as that by Russell and colleagues,[14] demonstrated significantly higher infection rates in tibial shaft fractures treated with primary closure (20%) compared with the infection rate of those patients treated with delayed primary closure at 5 days to 7 days (3%).[14] The study, however, compares 2 heterogeneous groups in terms of fracture severity, and comparisons are thus difficult to perform. In contrast, DeLong and colleagues[15] reported on 119 open fractures where a majority of grades II and III injuries were treated with primary closure. With comparable groups, they found no difference in infection rate (7%) when primary versus delayed closure was evaluated.

Perhaps the most rigorous débridement protocol was published by Lenarz and colleagues.[16] Patients were taken to the operating room for débridement and fixation, with cultures taken at the time of each débridement. If cultures became positive within 48 hours, patients underwent serial débridements until cultures were negative and closure could be obtained. Cultures found positive after 48 hours were treated with watchful waiting and antibiotics. With this protocol 422 open fractures of both upper and lower extremity (breakdown not stated in the study) were treated and time to definitive closure for grade I was 0.76 days, grade II 14.47 days, and grade III 18.5 days. The overall average rate of deep infection was 4.3%; however, grade IIIb fracture had a

10.6% infection rate and the grade IIIc fractures had a 20% infection rate. Thus, it remains true that infection rate is more likely due to the condition of the soft tissue envelope that the time to wound closure.[16]

In the distal radius, there are few data to guide surgeons with regard to serial débridements for contaminated wounds. Extrapolating from studies in the lower extremity, the evidence certainly supports serial staged débridements until wounds are amenable to definitive fixation. The exception to the rule are Gustilo I open fractures of the distal radius. Several studies have demonstrated low infection rates in these injuries and suggest they can be managed in similar fashion to their closed counterparts.[5,8,17,18]

ROLE OF ANTIBIOTICS

The immediate administration of intravenous antibiotics on presentation has been considered the standard of care in the treatment of open fractures. A majority of the data supporting this treatment were derived from work completed approximately 3 decades ago by Gustilo and Anderson.[19] In their study, which included 673 open tibia fractures studied retrospectively and 352 open tibia fractures studied prospectively, standard administration of oxacillin-ampicillin prior to surgery and continued for 72 hours postoperatively resulted in an infection rate of 2.5% (decreased from their retrospective study). The investigators argued that because bacterial growth occurred in 70.3% of all wound cultures, the standard administration of a cephalosporin provided both prophylactic and therapeutic benefit in these patients.

Since that time, several levels I and II studies have demonstrated that antibiotics definitively reduce the risk of postoperative infections in open fractures by approximately 50%.[20–22] An often quoted study by Patzakis and Wilkins[23] advocates for the administration of antibiotics within 3 hours (4.7% infection rate if administered within 3 h vs 7.4% if administered after 3 h) yet no statistical comparison was made between these groups in this study. The current recommendation is to administer antibiotics as early as possible.

The choice of antibiotics has often followed the Gustilo grading system. Work done by numerous groups, including Patzakis and colleagues[24] and Gustilo,[25] demonstrated level I evidence that administration of a first-generation cephalosporin reduces the risk of postoperative infection after an open fracture (from 13.9% in controls to 2.3% in the cephalosporin group),[24,25] because it is active against a majority of gram-positive cocci, gram-negative rods, *Escherichia coli*, and *Klebsiella pneumonia*.

Broadening antibiotic coverage for increasingly severe/contaminated wounds has become common practice, despite scant evidence for support.[26] The addition of an aminoglycoside or third-generation cephalosporin for grades II and III fractures is based on the historically high rate of infection with gram-negative organisms.[27] The gram-negative organisms observed in these initial studies were organisms now considered nosocomial pathogens (such as *Pseudomonas aeruginosa*) as opposed to contaminants from the initial injury. Normal skin flora and *Staphylococcus aureus* remain the most commonly isolated bacteria from open fracture wounds.[28] Therefore, the administration of an aminoglycoside or third-generation cephalosporin is likely influencing the rate of nosocomial infection in the setting of delayed wound closure as opposed to preventing an infection based on initial bacterial contamination.

In one of the few studies to prospectively evaluate the role of broadening antibiotic coverage, Johnson and colleagues[29] determined that there was no statistical difference in infection rate when comparing a first-generation versus third-generation cephalosporin for grade II/III tibia fractures. Their protocol consisted of 48 hours of initial therapy followed by culture tailored antibiotic treatment (a practice that is not currently followed or recommended). Despite stating that the severity of infection was higher with first-generation cephalosporins, there was no statistical difference between the groups regarding infection rate. When deciding whether or not to broaden antibiotic coverage with an aminoglycoside, clinicians must be mindful of the patient's renal function. Case reports exist detailing acute-onset renal failure after administration of either tobramycin or gentamycin calling into question their safety. Recently, however, several studies have shown that administration of an aminoglycoside in the initial 24-hour period after presentation for open fracture is safe and efficacious in reducing infection rate (provided renal function is normal at baseline).[30,31]

The addition of a high-dose penicillin has been advocated in the setting of gross contamination with soil or a farming injury with the goal of preventing gas gangrene. Similar to the administration of an aminoglycoside or third generation cephalosporin in grade II fractures, the evidence to support this practiced is lacking. In one of the earliest randomized controlled trials evaluating efficacy of antibiotic prophylaxis for open fractures, Patzakis[24] observed 2 cases of gas gangrene in the placebo group and thus advocated for routine administration of penicillin for anaerobic coverage. More recent work has shown that *Clostridium perfringens* is usually susceptible to first generation cephalosporins, suggesting that the administration of high dose penicillin is unnecessary.[32]

The optimal duration of antibiotic treatment of open fractures remains unclear (even for high-grade II/III injuries). Level I evidence fails to demonstrate a benefit to antibiotic duration greater than 24 hours after initial irrigation and débridement for grade I or II fractures and for 24 hours after coverage in grade III fractures.[33] Prolonged administration of broad spectrum antibiotics (3–5 d vs 24 h) has been shown an independent predictor of increased hospital stay, incidence of multidrug resistant infections, and mortality.[34] In the largest series of open distal radius fractures to date, Glueck and colleagues[3] evaluated 42 fractures (24 Gustilo I, 10 Gustilo II, and 8 Gustilo III) demonstrating an overall infection of 7%. All patients underwent operative débridement within 24 hours with serial débridement as deemed necessary by the operative surgeon as well as addition of antibiotics and tetanus prophylaxis according to standard to care at their institution. Subgroup analysis showed that it was the severity (extensive contamination with mud and soil) and type of contamination (fecal) not the time to débridement or Gustilo grade that determined infection rate.[3]

SURGICAL FIXATION

To date, the type of surgical fixation remains a matter of surgeon preference. Although some surgeons prefer definitive internal fixation at the index procedure, others use percutaneous techniques or temporary external fixation. Given the rare nature of these injuries, most clinical series include patients treated with a variety of different fixation methods making definitive conclusions difficult. MacKay and colleagues[18] compared a group of 18 open fractures treated with early débridement and fixation to 18 closed controls who were treated surgically. Types of fixation included a mixture of external fixation, percutaneous wiring, volar locked plates, and dorsal plates. Among the 2 groups, demographics and fracture type were similar, as were outcomes at 1 year. Range of motion, complications, strength, and patient-based outcome surveys demonstrated no difference in the 2 groups. These outcomes agree with data from prior studies with a nonunion rate of nearly one-third, whereas the investigators theorized that the increased soft tissue stripping and subsequent fracture devitalization may be identified as significant risk factors for nonunion independent of fixation strategy.

Kurylo and colleagues[2] reported on 32 patients with open injuries treated with external fixation, internal fixation, and staged internal fixation. They reported no infections in those treated with immediate internal fixation and concluded that immediate open reduction and internal fixation with plates may be safe in grades I and II injuries. Similarly, Glueck and colleagues[3] found that type of fixation was not a significant predictor of infection in their series of 42 patients. Kim and Park[17] treated 20 consecutive low-grade injuries with volar plates and compared them with 40 closed injuries. They found no difference in infection rate or in outcomes and 1 year after injury.

Based on the limited data, basic principles of operative fixation should prevail in either closed or open injuries, with the type of fixation chosen based strongly on the fracture pattern as opposed to a scoring system. In instances of heavy contamination, however, verification of débridement of devitalized tissue and foreign material is mandatory prior to proceeding with any method of fixation. Additionally, in those circumstances where the fixation technique may interfere with soft tissue management or would be at high risk for subsequent erosion or exposure, alternate techniques should be considered.

OUTCOMES AND COMPLICATIONS

Given the infrequent nature of these injuries, only a handful of studies have been published reporting the clinical outcomes of open distal radius fractures (**Table 3**). Rozental and colleagues[5] documented an average Disabilities of the Arm, Shoulder and Hand (DASH) score of 33 in a cohort of 18 patients. As expected, increasing injury severity by Gustilo classification was associated with a greater number of poor results and postoperative complications. Kaufman and colleagues[8] evaluated 21 patients with open fractures over the age of 60 and reported an arc of motion of 89° and an average QuickDASH score of 17.4, indicating minimal disability of the upper extremity. MacKay and colleagues[18] compared a group of 18 open fractures treated with early fixation with a group of 18 controls and found no difference in radiographic union, range of motion, or DASH scores. Kim and Park[17] reported on a group of low-grade open injuries treated with volar plates

Table 3
Summary of currently available studies reporting outcomes after open distal radius fractures

Author	Patients (N)	Gustilo Grade	Treatment	Infection Rate	Complication Rate	DASH Score
Rozental et al,[5] 2002	18	I: 9 II: 3 III: 6	Ex-fix: 15 Percutaneous: 2 ORIF: 1	8/18 (44%)	11/18 (61%)	33
Glueck et al,[3] 2009	42	I: 24 II: 10 III: 8	Ex-fix: 24 Staged sx-fix/ conversion to ORIF: 7 ORIF: 6 Percutaneous: 2 Casting: 3	3/42 (7%)	NA	NA
Kurylo et al,[2] 2011	32	I: 19 II: 11 III: 3	Ex-fix: 20 Staged ex-fix/ conversion to ORIF: 7 ORIF: 5	0/32 (0%)	8/32 (25%)	NA
Kim & Park,[17] 2013	20	I: 11 II: 9 III: 0	ORIF: 20	2/20 (10%)	5/20 (25%)	23
MacKay et al,[18] 2013	18	I: 11 II: 6 III: 1	Ex-fix: 6 ORIF: 12	1/18 (5%)	13/18 (72%)	13
Kaufman et al,[8] 2014	21	I: 12 II: 6 III: 3	Ex-fix: 3 ORIF: 18	1/21 (5%)	6/21 (29%)	17.4

Abbreviations: Ex-fix, external fixation; NA, not available; ORIF, open reduction internal fixation.

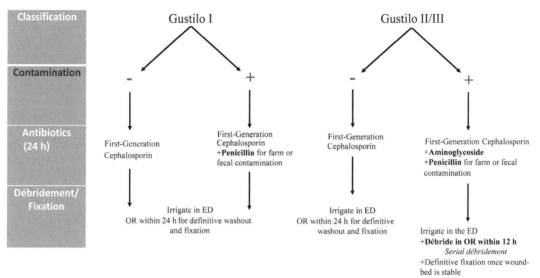

Fig. 1. Decision tree for comprehensive management of open distal radius fractures. ED, emergency department; OR, operating room.

and found similar DASH scores and range of motion at 1 year compared with a closed fracture comparison group.

Complications among open injuries in these studies included infections, loss of reduction, nonunion, and complex regional pain syndrome. Again, more complex injuries are consistently associated with a higher rate of postoperative complications. Additionally, surgeons should be aware of the consideration that an open fracture may carry an associated increased risk of nonunion that may require bone grafting; revision surgery may be more frequent in this group.

The most salient point from these studies is that low-grade open distal radius fractures were associated with better outcomes and fewer complications, leading the authors to conclude that grade I open injuries behave more like their closed counterparts whereas grades II and III injuries have a guarded prognosis.

SUMMARY AND TREATMENT RECOMMENDATIONS

Open distal radius fractures are rare injuries and current literature consists entirely of small patient cohorts with a wide spectrum of injury severity. Although there may be limited evidence to guide management and treatment of these complicated injuries, the authors' preferred treatment algorithm is summarized in **Fig. 1**.

The initial evaluation necessitates a thorough irrigation, antibiotics, tetanus prophylaxis, and immobilization. The authors recommend assessing the degree of contamination in addition to the Gustilo score and level of soft tissue injury before deciding on the optimal management. Although low-grade injuries with small soft tissue defects can be treated with débridement and definitive fixation, high-grade and contaminated injuries may require serial débridements and temporary fixation. The type of operative fixation is dictated by the fracture pattern and the degree of soft tissue injury. Additionally, surgeons should be aware that an open fracture may carry an increased risk of nonunion that may require revision, and operative planning should include this consideration.

The authors' preference is to treat these injuries with definitive internal fixation whenever possible, because secondary operations for fracture fixation may be associated with an increased complication and revision rate. Surgeons should be aware that complex injury patterns carry a high risk of postoperative complications and should counsel their patients accordingly. Lastly, most grade I injuries can be treated like their closed counterparts with limited débridement and fixation and can expect excellent postoperative outcomes.

REFERENCES

1. Jawa A. Open fractures of the distal radius. J Hand Surg Am 2010;35(8):1348–50.
2. Kurylo JC, Axelrad TW, Tornetta P 3rd, et al. Open fractures of the distal radius: the effects of delayed debridement and immediate internal fixation on infection rates and the need for secondary procedures. J Hand Surg Am 2011;36(7):1131–4.

3. Glueck DA, Charoglu CP, Lawton JN. Factors associated with infection following open distal radius fractures. Hand (N Y) 2009;4:330–4.

4. Valderrama-Molina CO, Estrada-Castrillón M, Hincapie JA, et al. Intra- and interobserver agreement on the Oestern and Tscherne classification of soft tissue injury in periarticular lower-limb closed fractures. Colomb Med (Cali) 2014;45(4):173–8.

5. Rozental TD, Beredjiklian PK, Steinberg DR, et al. Open fractures of the distal radius. J Hand Surg Am 2002;27(1):77–85.

6. Friedrich PL. Die aseptische versorgung frischer wunden, unter mittheilung von thier-versuchen uber die auskeimungszeit von infectionserregern in frischen wunden. Arch Klin Chir 1898;57:288–310.

7. Ketonis C, Dwyer J, Ilyas AM. Timing of debridement and infection rates in open hand fractures of the hand: a systematic review. Hand (N Y) 2017;12(2):119–26.

8. Kaufman AM, Pensy RA, O'Toole RV, et al. Safety of immediate open reduction and internal fixation of geriatric open fractures of the distal radius. Injury 2014;45(3):534–9.

9. Khatod M, Botte MJ, Hoyt DB, et al. Outcomes in open tibia fractures: relationship between delay in treatment and infection. J Trauma 2003;55:949–54.

10. Al-Arabi YB, Nader M, Hamidian-Jahromi AR, et al. The effect of the timing of antibiotics and surgical treatment on infection rates in open long-bone fractures: a 9-year prospective study from a district general hospital. Injury 2007;38:900–5.

11. Swanson TV, Szabo RM, Anderson DD. Open hand fractures: prognosis and classification. J Hand Surg Am 1991;16(1):101–7.

12. Srour M, Inaba K, Okoye O, et al. Prospective evaluation of treatment of open fractures: effect of time to irrigation and debridement. JAMA Surg 2015;150:332–6.

13. Weber D, Dulai SK, Bergman J, et al. Time to initial operative treatment following open fracture does not impact development of deep infection: a prospective cohort study of 736 subjects. J Orthop Trauma 2014;28:613–9.

14. Russell GG, Henderson R, Arnett G. Primary or delayed closure for open tibial fractures. J Bone Joint Surg Am 1990;72B:125–8.

15. DeLong WG, Born CT, Wei SY, et al. Aggressive treatment of 119 open fracture wounds. J Trauma 1999;46:1049–54.

16. Lenarz CJ, Watson JT, Moed BR, et al. Timing of wound closure in open fractures based on cultures obtained after debridement. J Bone Joint Surg Am 2010;92:1921–6.

17. Kim JK, Park SD. Outcomes after volar plate fixation of low-grade open and closed distal radius fractures are similar. Clin Orthop Relat Res 2013;471(6):2030–5.

18. MacKay BJ, Montero N, Paksima N, et al. Outcomes following operative treatment of open fractures of the distal radius: a case control study. Iowa Orthop J 2013;33:12–8.

19. Gustilo RB, Anderson JT. Prevention of infection in the treatment of one thousand and twenty five open fractures of long bones: retrospective and prospective analyses. J Bone Joint Surg Am 1976;58(4):453–8.

20. Gosselin RA, Roberts I, Gillespie WJ. An- tibiotics for preventing infection in open limb fractures. Cochrane Database Syst Rev 2004;(1):CD003764.

21. Yun HC, Murray CK, Nelson KJ, et al. Infection after orthopaedic trauma: prevention and treatment. J Orthop Trauma 2016;30(Suppl 3):S21–6.

22. Lack WD, Karunakar MA, Angerame MR, et al. Type III open tibia fractures: immediate antibiotic prophylaxis minimizes infection. J Orthop Trauma 2015;29(1):1–6.

23. Patzakis MJ, Wilkins J. Factors influencing infection rate in open fracture wounds. Clin Orthop Relat Res 1989;243:36–40.

24. Patzakis MJ, Harvey JP Jr, Ivler D. The role of antibiotics in the management of open fractures. J Bone Joint Surg Am 1974;56(3):532–41.

25. Gustilo RB. Use of antimicrobial in the management of open fractures. Arch Surg 1979;114:805–8.

26. Wilkins J, Patzakis M. Choice and duration of antibiotics in open fractures. Orthop Clin North Am 1991;22(3):433–7.

27. Gustilo RB, Mendoza RM, Williams DN. Problems in the management of type III (severe) open fractures: a new classi cation of type III open fractures. J Trauma 1984;24(8):742–6.

28. Gustilo RB, Merkow RL, Templeman D. The management of open fractures. J Bone Joint Surg Am 1990;72(2):299–304.

29. Johnson KD, Bone LB, Scheinberg R. Severe open tibial fractures: a study protocol. J Orthop Trauma 1988;2(3):175–80.

30. Pannell WC, Banks K, Hahn J, et al. Antibiotic related acute kidney injury in patients treated for open fractures. Injury 2016;47(3):653–7.

31. Tessier JM, Moore B, Putty B, et al. Prophylactic gentamicin is not associated with acute kidney injury in patients with open fractures. Surg Infect (Larchmt) 2016;17(6):720–3.

32. Hauser CJ, Adams CA Jr, Eachempati SR. Council of the Surgical Infection Society. Surgical Infection Society guideline. Pro- phylactic antibiotic use in open fractures: an evidence-based guideline. Surg Infect (Larchmt) 2006;7(4):379–405.

33. Dellinger EP, Caplan ES, Weaver LD, et al. Duration of preventive antibiotic administration for open extremity fractures. Arch Surg 1988;123(3):333–9.

34. Velmahos GC, Toutouzas KG, Sarkisyan G, et al. Severe trauma is not an excuse for prolonged antibiotic prophylaxis. Arch Surg 2002;137(5):537–42.

Hand Compartment Syndrome

Aaron J. Rubinstein, MD, Irfan H. Ahmed, MD, Michael M. Vosbikian, MD*

KEYWORDS

- Compartment syndrome • Contracture • Fasciotomy • Hand trauma • Intracompartmental pressure

KEY POINTS

- Compartment syndrome is the result of a cascade of events leading to poor tissue perfusion and necrosis, which may lead to loss of limb or life.
- Both subjective findings and objective intracompartmental pressure measurements aid in the diagnosis of this condition.
- Minimizing the time to surgical decompression in a patient diagnosed with compartment syndrome is critical to optimize patient outcome.
- Adequate decompression of the 10 anatomic compartments of the hand is necessary at the time of fasciotomy.
- The sequelae of a missed or mistreated compartment syndrome can lead to poor outcomes plagued by contracture and functional disability of the hand.

INTRODUCTION

Acute compartment syndrome (ACS) is a potentially devastating condition seen across orthopedic specialties. This entity can be defined as a pathologic condition in which elevated interstitial pressure in a compartment bound by fascia results in a cascade of events that leads to vascular compromise, tissue ischemia, and necrosis. Depending on the severity of the particular case, the impact on the patient may range from minimal functional deficits to loss of limb or life.[1–4] For this reason, not only is it of paramount importance to make the diagnosis, but to make it quickly, as many studies have shown irreversible changes being directly related to elapsed time.[5–9] In addition, the medicolegal ramifications of timely treatment in compartment syndrome cannot be understated.[1,2]

The diagnosis of ACS is often a challenging one. The patients are often in an altered mental state or medically unstable, which can result in an unreliable or unobtainable subjective history and examination.[4,7,9–12] For this reason, much attention has been directed toward the objective measurement of the interstitial pressure in the affected compartment. Arterial line manometers as well as commercially available devices are available and have been validated as diagnostic adjuncts in the hospital setting.[2–4,6,8,13–15]

However, even in the presence of these subjective and objective data, the diagnosis can be unclear. Numerous studies have sought to determine a concrete set of criteria for diagnosis based on pressure thresholds.[10,16,17] However, there is still no absolute consensus. For this reason, clinical vigilance and acumen are crucial to optimizing patient outcomes.

HISTORICAL PERSPECTIVE

Richard Von Volkmann first described compartment syndrome as "… a quick and massive disintegration of the contractile substance and the

Department of Orthopaedic Surgery, Rutgers University, New Jersey Medical School, 140 Bergen Street, D-1610, Newark, NJ 07103, USA
* Corresponding author.
E-mail address: vosbikmm@njms.rutgers.edu

Hand Clin 34 (2018) 41–52
https://doi.org/10.1016/j.hcl.2017.09.005
0749-0712/18/© 2017 Elsevier Inc. All rights reserved.

effect of the ensuing reaction and degeneration" in 1881.[18] After witnessing limb paralysis and subsequent contracture in the setting of prolonged compression from constrictive dressings, Volkmann[18] was the first to contend that compartment syndrome is a myogenic condition due to prolonged ischemia, later attributed to an ischemic threshold in excess of more than 6 hours. His hypothesis was contrary to the dogma of his contemporaries, which at the time, felt as if the condition was the sequelae of a compressive neuropathy.

Since that time, much effort has been invested in studying the nature and consequences of ACS. Coined by Bywaters and Beall[19] in 1941, the term, "the crush syndrome," later revised to "ischemic muscle necrosis" was used to describe the extremity injuries and rapid systemic decompensation that occurred in the victims of the London bombings in World War II. These findings were consistently found in those who had experienced prolonged external compression or crush injury of an extremity, thus validating Volkmann's[18] hypothesis.[19] Further studies by Bentley and Jeffreys[20] in the coal mining population noted similar findings. These works demonstrated that compartment syndrome, although initially localized, carries a true potential for the rapid development of shock and multisystem organ failure when left untreated, resulting in significant morbidity or mortality.[20]

Due to the severity of this condition and the highly varied etiologies of compartment syndrome, research began to focus on risk factors and diagnostic criteria. In her pivotal work, McQueen and colleagues[21] evaluated 164 patients with compartment syndrome over an 8-year period, noting that men younger than 35 years of age were at the highest risk. In their series, fracture was the most common cause of ACS in the upper extremity, with the distal radius most often implicated, followed by a traumatic injury without an associated fracture. Additionally, the presence of a bleeding disorder or anticoagulation was noted in 10% of the studied population.[21] This correlation has been seen in other series as well.[22]

Compartment syndrome of the hand is relatively rare, when compared with the lower extremity, but is associated with a multitude of underlying causes. Initially described by Bunnell and colleagues,[23] in 1948, it was deemed distinct from the characteristic Volkmann's ischemic contracture of the upper extremity, summarized as, "absolutely unrecoverable" pertaining to cases involving the hand when intrinsic releases were not released in a timely fashion. Since the description by Bunnell and colleagues,[23] many cases and small series pertaining to the treatment of hand compartment syndrome have been detailed in the literature, yet a paucity of large, concrete evidence still remains.

ANATOMY

The hand is commonly described as being composed of 10 fascially bound myotendinous compartments. Although anatomic studies suggest the presence of variability among individuals, the hand compartments are most often described as the thenar, hypothenar, adductor, and 7 interosseous compartments. Although technically at the wrist, the carpal canal is an area often involved in this process as well. Each of these compartments is bound by its own fascial envelope. With respect to the digits, despite the absence of discrete muscle bellies, the spaces created by the boundaries of Grayson and Cleland ligaments are often considered to be individual compartments.

The thenar compartment lies volar and in the most radial position, bound by the thenar fascia. Its components include the muscle bellies of the thenar intrinsic muscles: the opponens pollicis, abductor pollicis brevis, and flexor pollicis brevis. These muscles are primarily innervated by the recurrent median nerve with some contribution from the ulnar nerve. DiFelice and colleagues,[24] in a cadaveric injection study, focused on the myofascial compartments of 21 cadaveric hands by evaluating postinjection anatomic cross-sections to better delineate anatomic nuances. Interestingly, 52% of thenar compartment specimens were found to contain 2 or more discrete myofascial spaces. This study served to show that hand compartment anatomy is variable and less consistent than found in the lower extremity, an anatomic subtlety to be accounted for in the clinical setting.[24]

The adductor compartment, shown to be a discrete compartment in 71% of the specimens evaluated by DiFelice and colleagues,[24] is composed solely of the adductor pollicis muscle. Its anatomic position is volar, located between the radial lumbricals and volar interossei of the first webspace. The innervation of the adductor originates from the motor branch of the ulnar nerve in the palm.[24]

Initially suggested to be discrete compartments by Halpern and colleagues,[25] the interosseous compartments are likely to be more heterogeneous than once thought. However, there is some debate regarding their variability and the clinical significance of the aforementioned anatomic variation. There are 4 dorsal and 3 interosseous muscles in the hand, each innervated by motor branches originating from the ulnar nerve. A combined compartment with the first dorsal interosseous muscle and adductor compartments was noted in 19% of specimens in the study by DiFelice and colleagues.[24] The remaining interosseous compartments demonstrated increasing variability, with communication found between the dorsal and volar components in as many as 57% of the specimens.[24] Guyton and colleagues[26] challenged the notion that the dorsal and volar interossei occupy distinct anatomic compartments with a real-time computed tomography contrast injection study focused on the second dorsal interosseous compartment while monitoring changes in intracompartmental pressure. The investigators found that contrast material communicated with both the first and second volar interossei in all specimens despite second dorsal intracompartmental pressures being below 15 mm Hg. These findings indicate that although fascial membranes may separate the volar and dorsal interossei, they may be rendered incompetent at relatively low pressures, and their clinical significance is less clear in the setting of ACS.

The final compartment, the hypothenar compartment, is located most ulnar and contains the hypothenar intrinsic musculature: the opponens digiti minimi, flexor digiti minimi, and abductor digiti minimi, all of which receive ulnar innervation. The hypothenar compartment has been demonstrated to have the most variable anatomy, with 76% of specimens having 2 or more discrete subcompartments.[24]

The carpal canal consists of the anatomic region bound by the transverse carpal ligament volarly, the scaphoid tubercle and trapezium radially, the hook of the hamate and pisiform ulnarly, and the proximal carpal row covered by the extrinsic carpal ligaments dorsally. It contains the tendons of the flexor digitorum superficialis, flexor digitorum profundus, flexor pollicis longus, and the median nerve. Increases in pressure within the carpal canal secondary to injury or insult can result in acute carpal tunnel syndrome, which presents with increasing pain and paresthesias secondary to the compressive effects on the median nerve at this level, which can progress to permanent nerve dysfunction.[5,9,27–29]

PATHOPHYSIOLOGY

Compartment syndrome occurs when pressure within a bounded myofascial space exceeds the ability for tissues to receive adequate inflow for perfusion. This inflow deficit results in the development of ischemia and cellular changes, leading to apoptosis on the cellular level. This is most often secondary to direct increases in compartment pressure by a pathologic process such a fracture or an intracompartmental bleed, or due to external compression, as is seen with tight constrictive dressings or casts.[2,7,10,30–32] The underlying pathophysiology is complex and multiple theories have evolved from clinical observation as well as laboratory studies (**Fig. 1**).

Early work from Ashton proposed a critical closing pressure.[33] This pressure is defined as the threshold at which vessel collapse occurs from compression exceeding a vessel's intraluminal pressure. The investigator states that vessel wall tension (T_c) represents a constricting force composed of both passive vessel wall elasticity and active vessel muscular tone. Wall tension is related to transmural pressure, or the difference between intravascular pressure and interstitial pressure, by the law of Laplace: $P_{TM} = T_c/r$, where r is the vessel radius. Critical closure occurs when the P_{TM} is sufficiently low and the vessel collapses under instability. This can occur when the active vessel tone increases significantly or when the P_{TM} is decreased secondary to depleted intravascular volume or increased surrounding interstitial pressure. Because this theory relates to both the muscle tone and caliber of the vessel, the investigator proposed that the arteriole, with its muscular wall and small radius, would be expected to be the first vessel subject to critical closing.[33]

Later works evaluating the microvascular anatomy of injured tissue have disputed Ashton's early findings. Schaser and colleagues[34] created a closed soft tissue injury in a murine model with the goal of evaluating microvascular perfusion, edema, and intramuscular pressure. In their model, the most pronounced changes in microvascular permeability were noted in the venules following the injury. Although compartment syndrome was not directly created in this study, these findings suggest that, in the setting of trauma, the etiology of compartment syndrome may be related to venule diameter. They proposed that these venules are the most responsive to interstitial pressure changes, not the arterioles as was previously suggested.

In the current literature, the prevailing theory for the development of compartment syndrome hinges on the "arterio-venous pressure gradient differential" model. This concept states that an increase in intracompartmental pressure results in an external compression of the microvasculature within the compartment first. Efferent capillaries and venules, with their small diameter and lack of intramural musculature, are the most sensitive to pressure changes, and will begin to collapse first. As venous congestion and back pressure ensue

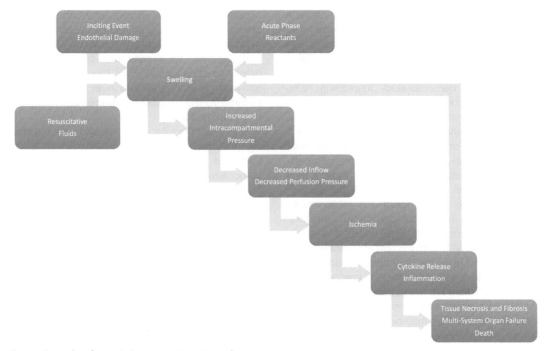

Fig. 1. Cascade of events in compartment syndrome.

from compression of the outflow system, a diminished arterio-venous gradient is generated. This disruption of the gradient leads to a decrease in local perfusion pressure and leads to ischemia. A secondary effect of this congestion is an increase in the pressure exerted on the vessel walls, causing an extravasation of fluid into the extravascular space. This so-called, "third-spacing" results in increased tissue edema and interstitial pressure generating a positive feedback loop, which increases external pressure on the intracompartmental vasculature.[2,5,7,9,34] Lymphatics, which theoretically assist with outflow and decompression, fail rapidly as intracompartmental pressures rise, thus having a negligible effect on the intracompartmental pressure.[8,35]

As this cascade continues to perpetuate, a critical threshold for tissue ischemia is reached as inflow is no longer able to meet the metabolic needs of the tissues. Dahn and colleagues,[32] in a 1967 study, concluded that blood flow to a region ceases when interstitial pressure reaches the diastolic pressure of the individual. As pressures reach this threshold, muscles are deprived of oxygen and metabolic supply. Changes in cellular metabolism result in the production of reactive oxidative species, such as xanthine oxidase, which damage endothelial cells, further increasing vascular permeability. This increase in permeability, as stated previously, leads to fluid leakage into the interstitial space, increasing external

pressure and decreasing tissue perfusion pressure.[2] Neutrophils and other inflammatory cells are drawn to the ischemic regions and release cytokines and chemical mediators from their own metabolism, which exacerbate the vascular permeability, further increasing interstitial pressure and perpetuating the cycle.[2,9,34–36]

PATHOLOGIC IMPLICATIONS

To ascertain the effects on peripheral nerve function in the setting of compartment syndrome, Gelberman and colleagues[37] developed an in vivo model to determine clinical effects. The investigators evaluated peripheral nerve function in humans while increasing the pressure exerted around the median nerve. Using direct, external compression of the carpal canal, they noted that at a tissue fluid pressure threshold of 40 to 50 mm Hg, sensory and motor function of the median nerve demonstrated partial to complete blockade. Thus, the investigators concluded that at this level, decompressive release is warranted.

Heppenstall and colleagues[38] sought to delineate the cellular effects of compartment syndrome in several studies using the mean arterial pressure (MAP) as a reference point. In a canine study, the effects of tissue ischemia by tourniquet occlusion were compared with the effects of ACS, produced by intracompartmental plasma infusion. It was noted that adenosine triphosphate (ATP) stores diminished more rapidly, and ischemic acidosis was more profound in the ACS group when compared with the tourniquet group. Secondarily, the ACS group was found to have a significantly slower time to recovery following pressure reversal than the tourniquet group. In a subsequent study, nuclear magnetic resonance spectroscopy and electron microscopy were used to evaluate the effect of varying tissue pressures on skeletal muscle metabolism in an in vivo canine ACS model. The study found that the difference between the MAP and intracompartmental pressure (delta P) was more closely associated with resultant metabolic changes rather than the absolute pressure of the intracompartmental space. The investigators suggest that a delta P of 30 mm Hg in normal muscle and 40 mm Hg in traumatized muscle as the threshold for metabolic derangement. This conclusion proposes that injured muscle has a lower threshold for developing compartment syndrome than healthy muscle, which speaks to the need for clinical vigilance in the trauma population.[17] McQueen and Court-Brown,[16] in their clinical series echoed this finding using a delta P of 30 mm Hg as their threshold to perform a decompressive fasciotomy. Their outcomes validated the canine study by Heppenstall and colleagues[17] in the human population.

Heckman and colleagues[39] also tried to determine the critical intracompartmental pressure at which irreversible muscle damage would occur. Using a plasma infusion model and a reference point of the diastolic blood pressure (DBP), rather than the MAP, compartment pressures were elevated to varying degrees for an 8-hour duration and compared with the DBP. Subsequent histologic sections were prepared and evaluated for signs of muscle injury, fibrosis, and infarction. The microscopic findings concluded that at a delta P of 20 mm Hg, histologic changes were first noted, and once the pressure reached a delta P of 10 mm Hg, irreversible tissue damage and muscle fibrosis was induced.

Although compartment syndrome clearly threatens limb function, a threat to the patient's life can also develop without appropriate, timely treatment. With prolonged muscle ischemia, myocyte necrosis and degradation ensue. The resultant release of myoglobin from apoptosis leads to increased renal stress and damage, leading to acute renal failure, and hyperkalemia. This hyperkalemia and other electrolyte derangements result in cardiac conduction abnormalities and possible arrhythmias leading to cardiac arrest. In addition to cardiac complications, shock can result from systemic exposure to proinflammatory cytokines and enzymes, which can culminate in multisystem organ failure.[7]

ETIOLOGIES

ACS can arise from any pathologic condition inducing an increase in the intracompartmental pressure within a fascially bound compartment. Fundamentally, this can be caused by a multitude of processes that result in a direct pressure increase or an external compression stimulus. In a pivotal study, McQueen and colleagues[21] found that fractures were the most common cause of ACS with 69% of all of their ACS cases occurring with a concomitant fracture.

However, the literature on ACS of the hand suggests that the etiologies and their incidence may not coincide with the rest of the upper extremity and lower extremity. Due to the low incidence of hand compartment syndrome, few large studies exist, thus most occurrences are presented as case reports or small case series. As such, reported cases demonstrate a wide range of underlying causes, including but not limited to, complications related to intravenous infiltrations, crush injuries, fractures, prolonged external compression, insect bites, stings, snake envenomation, high-pressure injections, infection, bleeding, and burns (**Box 1**).[5,10,22,25,35,40–44]

In one of the larger series, Ouellette and Kelly[10] conducted a retrospective review of 19 patients over a 5-year period, defining several characteristics of ACS of the hand. In a patient population ranging from 5 months to 67 years of age, there was a near even distribution of adults and children. Thirteen (68%) of these 19 cases were found to be iatrogenic in nature with intravenous line complications resulting in 11 cases and arterial line complications causing 2 cases. Other causes listed were a gunshot wound, a crush injury, and prolonged external compression in a patient admitted for a drug overdose. Of note, 15 of the 19 patients had an altered sensorium during ACS diagnosis, emphasizing the need for physician vigilance and the use of validated, objective intracompartmental measurement techniques for diagnosis when evaluating at-risk individuals.

EVALUATION AND DIAGNOSIS

A diagnosis of ACS can often be made using patient history and physical examination alone, with objective diagnostic studies used for confirmation or clarification in the setting of equivocal findings.[2–4,6–10,13,14,45] It is important to maintain a high degree of suspicion, when appropriate, as early delays in treatment can translate into debilitating consequences.[5–9,18]

Evaluation should begin with a thorough patient history. Even in the obtunded patient, an

---

Box 1
Etiologies of compartment syndrome

Traumatic
Fractures
Dislocations
Blunt trauma
Crush injuries
Penetrating/gunshot injuries
Burns
Envenomation
High-pressure injection

Medical
Infection
Bleeding disorders
Spontaneous hemorrhage
Rhabdomyolysis

Iatrogenic
Ischemia-reperfusion
Intravenous infiltration
Contrast extravasation
Constrictive dressings or casts
Arthroscopy
Prolonged pressure from positioning

Vascular
Arterial injury
Arterial puncture
Arterial catheterization
Venous occlusion

---

understanding of the mechanism of injury or history as obtained through a health care provider's report can appropriately serve to guide a clinical suspicion. One should ask about the mechanism of injury, the environment, if there was any entrapment, and about the sequence and timing of events, among other things. As previously discussed, compartment syndrome of the hand has been attributed to a variety of causes. However, complications relating to intravenous infusions, high-energy trauma, crush injury, or prolonged external compression should be evaluated with added caution.[5,10] With respect to patient factors, those with congenital or acquired coagulopathic states, or those taking blood thinners are at an elevated risk.

Classically, the "5 Ps," as described by Griffiths,[46] have been used to describe the clinical findings of compartment syndrome: pain, paresthesia, pallor, paralysis, and pulselessness. It should be noted, however, that these findings are more consistent with an arterial occlusion, set forth by Griffiths[46] on the belief that arterial spasm was the predominate cause of ACS.[47] As recent evidence has shown the more complex nature of ACS, these symptoms have been accepted as later findings, and are less commonly used, as their presence may be a harbinger of permanent damage. Sensory changes and paralysis will not manifest until at least 1 hour after a critical ischemic intracompartmental pressure is reached.[48] Currently, most clinicians will agree that increasing or disproportionate pain, often demonstrated by an increased analgesic requirement, is the most common early finding in ACS.[2,5,9,10] This is particularly important in the pediatric patient population.[7,49]

A detailed physical examination will further aid the clinician in diagnosis. A thorough inspection, palpation, and a neurovascular examination of the entire extremity should be performed. Ouellette and Kelly[10] noted that the most consistent physical examination finding in ACS of the hand was a tense, swollen hand with intrinsic minus posturing (extension of the metacarpophalangeal joints and flexion of the proximal and distal interphalangeal joints). Additionally, pain with passive stretch of the intracompartmental muscles has been shown to be the most sensitive finding of impending ischemic changes, which has been shown to occur with intracompartmental pressure increases from a baseline of 0 to 8 mm Hg to 30 to 40 mm Hg in a normotensive individual (**Fig. 2**).[48]

In the hand, specific compartments can be evaluated by different physical examination maneuvers: the dorsal and volar interossei can be evaluated by passively adducting and abducting the digits with the metacarpophalangeal (MP) joints in flexion and interphalangeal (IP) joints in extension, the so-called intrinsic plus position. The lumbrical musculature can be tested by passive extension at the MP joint while flexing the proximal IP joint. Thenar musculature can be evaluated by thumb adduction, thus stretching the abductor pollicus brevis. Conversely, the adductor compartment is tested by passive thumb abduction. Last, the hypothenar musculature is evaluated by passive adduction and extension of the small finger, thus putting the abductor digiti minimi and flexor digiti minimi in a stretched position.[2] With respect to increased pressure in the carpal canal, leading to acute carpal tunnel syndrome, the diagnosis is more clinical and marked by increasing pain and radial-sided acroparesthesias in the median nerve distribution.

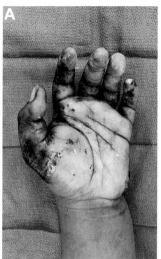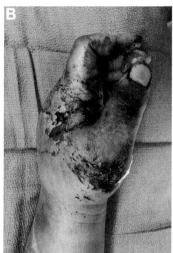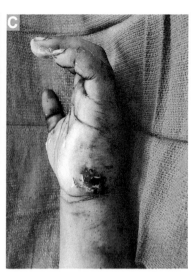

Fig. 2. (A–C) Clinical photographs of a patient with hand compartment syndrome. Note the loss of palmar concavity and intrinsic minus position.

As these physical examination findings are likely to occur before the onset of sensory paresthesias, which may blunt a patient's perception of pain, they serve as good clinical indicators for ACS, which in theory will manifest themselves earlier in the clinical course. Matsen and colleagues[50] evaluated the effects of increasing pressures on the peripheral nervous system, and noted a sequential loss of neurologic function beginning with light touch, then progressing to motor weakness before the dampening of painful stimuli and resultant anesthesia, which signifies severe nerve damage. This progressive conduction block occurs at a threshold between 40 and 50 mm Hg of pressure, as demonstrated by Gelberman and colleagues.[37]

Often, in obtunded or uncooperative patients, neurologic examination is unattainable, and clinicians are left to use digital palpation and pulse examination to help guide diagnosis. However, the literature has shown that neither of these findings are very sensitive for an accurate ACS diagnosis. Wong and colleagues,[4] in a cadaveric compartment syndrome model, evaluated the accuracy of digital palpation in a population of 17 orthopedic residents and attending physicians. The investigators found that the sensitivity and specificity of digital palpation of the thenar compartment was 49% and 79%, respectively. In the hypothenar compartment, the sensitivity and specificity of palpation were 62% and 83%, respectively. Both sensitivity and specificity were improved significantly to greater than 90% with use of a handheld manometer. Regarding pulse examination, absence of pulses is a less common finding, and indicative of a late diagnosis of ACS. Tissue ischemia and necrosis have been shown to occur even in setting of palpable distal pulses, and as such, the presence of pulses should not be the sole factor driving treatment decisions.[9]

To increase diagnostic accuracy, intracompartmental pressure measurement techniques are frequently used as a supportive tool in equivocal cases.[7] Many techniques have been described and validated for measuring pressure. Some of the more commonly used are the handheld compartment monitor, arterial line transducer, and a Whitesides apparatus.[4,6,13–15,45,51] Each apparatus can be used with various different needle types, including straight, side-port, and slit. It has been noted in the literature that these techniques vary in their accuracy of measurement. Boody and Wongworawat[13] compared the 9 possible permutations and noted that arterial line manometry was the most accurate technique when used with a slit catheter, whereas the handheld manometer with a side-port needle demonstrated the least constant bias in measured values. Straight needles were shown to be the least accurate, and the Whitesides apparatus showed an unacceptably high amount of variation and overestimation of intracompartmental pressure.[13] A study by Uliasz and colleagues[14] echoed the findings of Boody and Wongworawat,[13] demonstrating that the handheld manometer and intravenous pump techniques were both more accurate than the Whitesides device, whereas Moed and Thorderson[8] concluded that a simple needle technique consistently overestimated compartment pressures when compared with slit catheters and side-ported needles (**Figs. 3** and **4**).

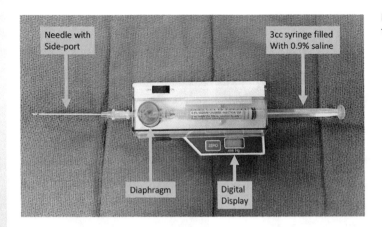

Fig. 3. Handheld intracompartmental pressure monitor.

To measure compartment pressures of the hand using a handheld manometer, the needle is inserted orthogonal to the skin and each compartment is evaluated separately. In addition, the hand should be at the level of the heart. The thenar and hypothenar compartments are entered at the junction of glabrous and nonglabrous skin. The dorsal interosseous compartments are measured 1 cm proximal to the metacarpal head and the needle advanced until the fascial compartment is entered. Advancing the needle approximately 5 mm deeper will allow the volar interosseous compartment to be measured. Entry on the radial side of the second metacarpal in the muscle of the webspace will allow assessment of the adductor compartment.[45] As mentioned previously, multiple studies have sought to evaluate the critical ischemic pressure for muscle tissue. Although some investigators suggest that an absolute pressure of 15 to 25 mm Hg with clinical symptoms or 25 mm Hg in asymptomatic patients be used as the cutoff for compartment syndrome, most clinicians will agree that fasciotomy is indicated when intracompartmental pressure in a single compartment is within 20 to 30 mm Hg of the patient's DBP (delta P).[5,10,12,45,51–53]

TREATMENT

In the event of suspected compartment syndrome, all constrictive dressings should be removed immediately and the extremity kept at the level of the heart. Elevating the extremity may lower the threshold for compartment syndrome from the decrease in tissue perfusion pressure caused by lowering the arterio-venous pressure gradient through the elevation-induced decrease in arterial inflow pressure.[2,6,9,50] If clinical suspicion is not high enough to pursue immediate treatment, serial neurovascular examinations and intracompartmental pressure measurements can be performed.

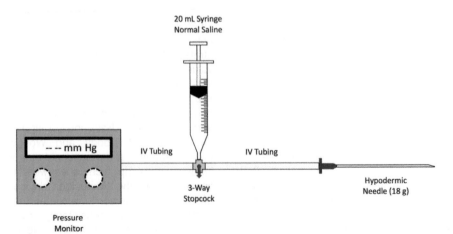

Fig. 4. Schematic of pressure monitoring set up.

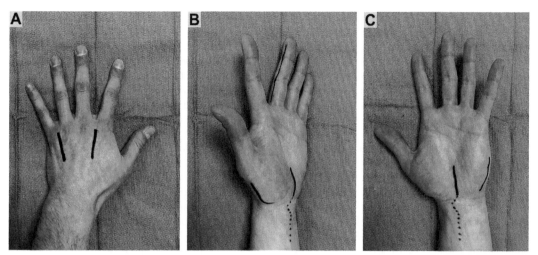

Fig. 5. (A–C) Incisions commonly used for release of hand compartments. (A) Dorsal incisions for release of interosseous and adductor compartments, (B) Incisions for release of the thenar compartment, carpal canal, and mid-axial decompression of the digit, (C) Incisions for release of the hypothenar compartment and carpal canal.

Once a diagnosis of ACS is made, the mainstay of treatment is a timely, decompressive fasciotomy. There is traditionally little role for nonoperative management of ACS, and delays in surgical intervention result in poorer outcomes.[5–9] The technique for release of the dorsal and volar interossei as well as the adductor compartment involves making separate longitudinal dorsal incisions over the second and fourth metacarpals. Dissection is carried down along the sides of each metacarpal, and the fascia is incised. Deeper dissection is continued along the radial aspect of

the second metacarpal to release the adductor compartment. A similar technique is used along the radial and ulnar side of each metacarpal to decompress the volar interossei. To release the thenar and hypothenar compartments, volar incisions are made at the glabrous non-glabrous junction radial to the first metacarpal and ulnar to the fifth metacarpal respectively to gain appropriate access for decompression. Necrotic tissue, if present, should be debrided during the decompression, as it will serve as a potential nidus of infection.[2,5,7,9]

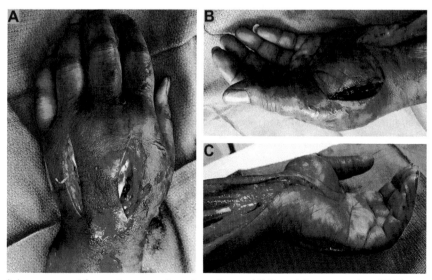

Fig. 6. Hand decompressed for acute compartment syndrome. (A) Dorsal decompression, (B) Thenar and carpal canal decompression, (C) Hypothenar and carpal canal decompression. (*Courtesy of* Katharine T. Criner-Woozley, MD, Philadelphia, PA.)

The carpal canal can be decompressed through a standard incision made along the radial axis of the ring finger, starting from the Kaplan cardinal line and working proximally the volar wrist crease. This can be extended more proximally into an extended carpal tunnel incision to increase the amount of median nerve decompression possible. Digital decompression, if indicated, is performed using midaxial incisions releasing the Cleland ligaments, taking caution to avoid the neurovascular bundles that can be retracted volarly (**Figs. 5** and **6**).[9]

After decompression, the wounds are typically left open and dressed with moist dressings, or a negative pressure wound therapy system. The hand should be splinted in a safe position of function, with 70 to 90° of flexion at the metacarpophalangeal joints and 0 to 10° of flexion at the proximal and distal interphalangeal joints, the so-called intrinsic plus position. The surgical wounds should be reevaluated every 2 to 3 days for infection until closure or other definitive coverage is permitted. Often, a split thickness skin graft is required to cover the remaining defects. Physical and occupational therapy exercises emphasizing early range of motion are implemented as early as possible to avoid contractures and functional deficits.[2,5]

One technique that can aid in the prevention or minimization of post-compartment syndrome contracture is external fixation of the first webspace. The multiplanar technique described by Harper and Iorio[54] uses half pins in the first and second metacarpals to hold the thumb maximally abducted postoperatively while the soft tissues heal. In their series of 5 patients (2 table saw injuries, 2 burn contractures, and 1 oncologic reconstruction), they found an average QuickDASH score of 35 and a Modern Activity Subjective Survey of 2007 score of 30, which heavily weights the use of the first webspace and thumb circumduction.[54] Similar success was found in a series by Acartürk and colleagues,[55] in the setting of preestablished thumb adduction contractures with wrist contractures. Their findings show that this technique can be effective both in the acute and reconstructive periods.

OUTCOMES AND COMPLICATIONS

The most morbid functional complication associated with ACS is intrinsic contracture. As muscle ischemia progresses to tissue necrosis, the muscle bellies become fibrotic and as a result, shorten, producing deformity consistent with contracture. The hand will assume an intrinsic minus position with the metacarpophalangeal joints in extension and the interphalangeal joints in flexion. In addition, the first webspace is contracted. With this posture, the prognosis for functional recovery is low. Due to the functional incapacitation from this sequelae, timing to treatment is critical. It has been shown that the time from diagnosis until fasciotomy is the single most important indicator of clinical outcome. Delays to decompression greater than 8 hours are consistent with irreversible, ischemic damage to muscle tissue.[7]

The current body of hand surgery literature on long term follow-up and functional outcomes of ACS of the hand is lacking. In the retrospective review conducted by Oulette and Kelly, the average follow-up period was 21 months. Four of the 19 patients in the study were deemed to have a poor result, with significant loss of hand function. In all instances, the time from diagnosis, not necessarily the onset of ACS, to treatment was prolonged, a period defined as more than 6 hours. In the 4 patients with a poor result, all were obtunded, 3 were children, and 2 eventually required an amputation. No correlation with level of intracompartmental pressure and functional outcome was found following fasciotomy. Contrary to prior conclusions regarding children having more favorable outcomes, follow-up data showed that 8 of 9 adults regained normal function of the hand, whereas only 5 of 8 children regained the same level of function as their adult counterparts. The investigators suggest that a communication barrier may play a role or alternatively, that the pediatric patients in their series were more in extremis.[10]

SUMMARY

ACS is a potentially devastating condition that is the result of a complex cascade that begins at an inciting event, and if not treated, leads to increased interstitial pressure, tissue necrosis, and cellular death that can result in loss of function, limb, or life. The potential etiologies are myriad, which require the clinician to have sound acumen and vigilance in making a timely diagnosis. Oftentimes, the patients are of an altered sensorium, thus objective measurements with commercially available or assembled pressure monitors are useful in equivocal cases. After the diagnosis is made, it is critical to expeditiously perform a decompressive fasciotomy of all involved compartments to halt the cascade and prevent the potential sequelae of an untreated compartment syndrome and maximize functional outcomes.

REFERENCES

1. Bhattacharyya T, Vrahas MS. The medical-legal aspects of compartment syndrome. J Bone Joint Surg Am 2004;86(4):864–8.

2. Seiler JG III, Olvey SP. Compartment syndromes of the hand and forearm. J Am Soc Surg Hand 2003; 3(4):184–98.

3. Mubarak SJ, Owen CA, Hargens AR, et al. Acute compartment syndromes: diagnosis and treatment with the aid of the wick catheter. J Bone Joint Surg Am 1978;60(8):1091–5.

4. Wong JC, Vosbikian MM, Dwyer JM, et al. Accuracy of measurement of hand compartment pressures: a cadaveric study. J Hand Surg Am 2015;40(4):701–6.

5. Oak NR, Abrams RA. Compartment syndrome of the hand. Orthop Clin North Am 2016;47(3):609–16.

6. Matsen FA, Winquist RA, Krugmire RB. Diagnosis and management of compartmental syndromes. J Bone Joint Surg Am 1980;62(2):286–91.

7. Prasarn ML, Ouellette EA. Acute compartment syndrome of the upper extremity. J Am Acad Orthop Surg 2011;19(1):49–58.

8. Moed BR, Thorderson PK. Measurement of intracompartmental pressure: a comparison of the slit catheter, side-ported needle, and simple needle. J Bone Joint Surg Am 1993;75(2):231–5.

9. Leversedge FJ, Moore TJ, Peterson BC, et al. Compartment syndrome of the upper extremity. J Hand Surg Am 2011;36(3):544–59 [quiz: 560].

10. Ouellette EA, Kelly R. Compartment syndromes of the hand. J Bone Joint Surg Am 1996;78(10):1515–22.

11. Shuler FD, Dietz MJ. Physicians' ability to manually detect isolated elevations in leg intracompartmental pressure. J Bone Joint Surg Am 2010;92(2):361–7.

12. Codding JL, Vosbikian MM, Ilyas AM. Acute compartment syndrome of the hand. J Hand Surg Am 2015;40(6):1213–6 [quiz: 1216].

13. Boody AR, Wongworawat MD. Accuracy in the measurement of compartment pressures: a comparison of three commonly used devices. J Bone Joint Surg Am 2005;87(11):2415–22.

14. Uliasz A, Ishida JT, Fleming JK, et al. Comparing the methods of measuring compartment pressures in acute compartment syndrome. Am J Emerg Med 2003;21(2):143–5.

15. Hammerberg EM, Whitesides TE Jr, Seiler JG III. The reliability of measurement of tissue pressure in compartment syndrome. J Orthop Trauma 2012; 26(1):24–31 [discussion: 32].

16. McQueen MM, Court-Brown CM. Compartment monitoring in tibial fractures. The pressure threshold for decompression. J Bone Joint Surg Br 1996;78(1): 99–104.

17. Heppenstall RB, Sapega AA, Scott R, et al. The compartment syndrome. An experimental and clinical study of muscular energy metabolism using phosphorus nuclear magnetic resonance spectroscopy. Clin Orthop Relat Res 1988;(226):138–55.

18. Volkmann RV. The classic: ischaemic muscle paralyses and contractures. Clin Orthop Relat Res 2007; 456:20–1.

19. Bywaters EG, Beall D. Crush injuries with impairment of renal function. Br Med J 1941;1(4185): 427–32.

20. Bentley G, Jeffreys TE. The crush syndrome in coal miners. J Bone Joint Surg Br 1968;50(3): 588–94.

21. McQueen MM, Gaston P, Court-Brown CM. Acute compartment syndrome. Who is at risk? J Bone Joint Surg Br 2000;82(2):200–3.

22. Ilyas AM, Wisbeck JM, Shaffer GW, et al. Upper extremity compartment syndrome secondary to acquired factor VIII inhibitor. A case report. J Bone Joint Surg Am 2005;87(7):1606–8.

23. Bunnell S, Doherty EW, Curtis RM. Ischemic contracture, local, in the hand. Plast Reconstr Surg (1946) 1948;3(4):424–33.

24. DiFelice A Jr, Seiler JG III, Whitesides TE Jr. The compartments of the hand: an anatomic study. J Hand Surg Am 1998;23(4):682–6.

25. Halpern AA, Greene R, Nichols T, et al. Compartment syndrome of the interosseous muscles: early recognition and treatment. Clin Orthop Relat Res 1979;140:23–5.

26. Guyton GP, Shearman CM, Saltzman CL. Compartmental divisions of the hand revisited. Rethinking the validity of cadaver infusion experiments. J Bone Joint Surg Br 2001;83(2):241–4.

27. Bauman TD, Gelberman RH, Mubarak SJ, et al. The acute carpal tunnel syndrome. Clin Orthop Relat Res 1981;(156):151–6.

28. Szabo RM. Acute carpal tunnel syndrome. Hand Clin 1998;14(3):419–29, ix.

29. Tosti R, Ilyas AM. Acute carpal tunnel syndrome. Orthop Clin North Am 2012;43(4):459–65.

30. Ashton H. Effect of inflatable plastic splints on blood flow. Br Med J 1966;2(5527):1427–30.

31. Aprahamian C, Gessert G, Bandyk DF, et al. MAST-associated compartment syndrome (MACS): a review. J Trauma 1989;29(5):549–55.

32. Dahn I, Lassen NA, Westling H. Blood flow in human muscles during external pressure or venous stasis. Clin Sci 1967;32(3):467–73.

33. Ashton H. Critical closure in human limbs. Br Med Bull 1963;19(2):149–54.

34. Schaser KD, Vollmar B, Menger MD, et al. In vivo analysis of microcirculation following closed soft-tissue injury. J Orthop Res 1999;17(5):678–85.

35. Sawyer JR, Kellum EL, Creek AT, et al. Acute compartment syndrome of the hand after a wasp sting: a case report. J Pediatr Orthop B 2010; 19(1):82–5.

36. Amsdell SL, Hammert WC. High-pressure injection injuries in the hand: current treatment concepts. Plast Reconstr Surg 2013;132(4):586e–91e.

37. Gelberman RH, Szabo RM, Williamson RV, et al. Tissue pressure threshold for peripheral nerve viability. Clin Orthop Relat Res 1983;(178):285–91.

38. Heppenstall RB, Scott R, Sapega A, et al. A comparative study of the tolerance of skeletal muscle to ischemia. Tourniquet application compared with acute compartment syndrome. J Bone Joint Surg Am 1986;68(6):820–8.

39. Heckman MM, Whitesides TE, Grewe SR, et al. Histologic determination of the ischemic threshold of muscle in the canine compartment syndrome model. J Orthop Trauma 1993;7(3):199–210.

40. Egro FM, Jaring MRF, Khan AZ. Compartment syndrome of the hand: beware of innocuous radius fractures. Eplasty 2014;14:46–51.

41. McKnight AJ, Koshy JC, Xue AS, et al. Pediatric compartment syndrome following an insect bite: a case report. Hand (N Y) 2011;6(3):337–9.

42. Werman H, Rancour S, Nelson R. Two cases of thenar compartment syndrome from blunt trauma. J Emerg Med 2013;44(1):85–8.

43. Sharma R, Rao RB, Chu J. Compartment syndrome of the hand from prolonged immobilization secondary to drug overdose. J Emerg Med 2013;44(4):845–6.

44. Belzunegui T, Louis CJ, Torrededia L, et al. Extravasation of radiographic contrast material and compartment syndrome in the hand: a case report. Scand J Trauma Resusc Emerg Med 2011;19(1):9.

45. Lipschitz AH, Lifchez SD. Measurement of compartment pressures in the hand and forearm. J Hand Surg Am 2010;35(11):1893–4.

46. Griffiths DL. Volkmann's ischaemic contracture. Br J Surg 1940;28(110):239–60.

47. Klenerman L. The evolution of the compartment syndrome since 1948 as recorded in the JBJS (B). J Bone Joint Surg Br 2007;89(10):1280–2.

48. Whitesides T, Heckman M. Acute compartment syndrome: Update on diagnosis and treatment. J Am Acad Orthop Surg 1996;4(4):209–18.

49. Bae DS, Kadiyala RK, Waters PM. Acute compartment syndrome in children: contemporary diagnosis, treatment, and outcome. J Pediatr Orthop 2001;21(5):680–8.

50. Matsen FA, Mayo KA, Krugmire RB, et al. A model compartmental syndrome in man with particular reference to the quantification of nerve function. J Bone Joint Surg Am 1977;59(5):648–53.

51. Whitesides TE, Haney TC, Morimoto K, et al. Tissue pressure measurements as a determinant for the need of fasciotomy. Clin Orthop Relat Res 1975;(113):43–51.

52. Matava MJ, Whitesides TE Jr, Seiler JG III, et al. Determination of the compartment pressure threshold of muscle ischemia in a canine model. J Trauma 1994;37(1):50–8.

53. Chandraprakasam T, Kumar RA. Acute compartment syndrome of forearm and hand. Indian J Plast Surg 2011;44(2):212–8.

54. Harper CM, Iorio ML. Prevention of thumb web space contracture with multiplanar external fixation. Tech Hand Up Extrem Surg 2016;20(3):91–5.

55. Acartürk TO, Ashok K, Lee WPA. The use of external skeletal fixation to facilitate the surgical release of wrist flexion and thumb web space contractures. J Hand Surg Am 2006;31(10):1619–25.

Forearm Compartment Syndrome
Evaluation and Management

Justin M. Kistler, MD[a,*], Asif M. Ilyas, MD[b],
Joseph J. Thoder, MD[a]

KEYWORDS

- Compartment syndrome • Forearm trauma • Volkmann • Upper extremity trauma • Fasciotomy

KEY POINTS

- Compartment syndrome is largely a clinical diagnosis and requires a careful history and physical examination.
- Compartment syndrome hallmarks have been the 5 Ps: pain out of proportion, pallor, paresthesias, paralysis, and pulselessness. Pain out of proportion and pain with passive stretching of the fingers are considered the first and most sensitive signs of compartment syndrome in an awake patient.
- In an obtunded patient, a compartment pressure measurement within 30 mm Hg of the diastolic blood pressure and/or an absolute pressure greater than 30 mm Hg is considered diagnostic for compartment syndrome.
- Adequate decompression of the forearm requires fascial release of both the dorsal and volar compartments, with the volar compartment best released from the carpal tunnel distally to across the lacertus fibrosus proximally.
- Fasciotomy wounds must be assessed every 48 hours to 72 hours and additional soft tissue coverage procedures for wound closure are common.

INTRODUCTION

Compartment syndrome of the forearm is an uncommon but well recognized diagnosis that can lead to significant morbidity and mortality if not diagnosed and treated early in the clinical course. Compartment syndrome is an increase in pressure within fascial compartments that can lead to decreased tissue perfusion. Compartment syndrome of the forearm typically presents with swelling of the forearm and patients complain of pain and difficulty with hand and wrist motion, particularly with passive motion. It may also be accompanied with paresthesias of the hand depending on the clinical course. The compartment syndrome may or may not be preceded by fracture or traumatic injury.

There are a variety of causes, both traumatic and nontraumatic, that can lead to forearm compartment syndrome, which can make the diagnosis and clinical decision-making process extremely complex. One of the most common causes reported are fractures of the forearm, including both diaphyseal forearm fractures and fractures of the distal radius.[1] Elliot and Johnstone[2] reported that 18% of all forearm

Disclosure Statement: The authors did not receive any compensation nor have any financial conflicts with the production of this article.
[a] Department of Orthopedic Surgery and Sports Medicine, Temple University, 3401 N. Broad Street, 5th Floor Boyer Pavilion, Philadelphia, PA 19104, USA; [b] Department of Orthopedic Surgery, Rothman Institute at Thomas Jefferson University, 925 Chestnut, Philadelphia, PA 19107, USA
* Corresponding author.
E-mail address: Justin.kistler2@tuhs.temple.edu

hand.theclinics.com

compartment syndromes were caused by fractures of the forearm. In contrast, it was reported that only 23% of all forearm compartment syndromes are caused by some form of soft tissue trauma not involving fractures. There are more unusual causes of forearm compartment syndrome, including reperfusion injury, angioplasty or angiography, intravenous line extravasations, injection of illicit drugs, coagulopathies or bleeding disorders, hematoma in patients treated with anticoagulants, and even insect bites.[1,3–11]

The diagnosis of compartment syndrome is predominantly clinical, but several techniques have been described and studied. Yet, controversy persists on the best diagnostic techniques. Regardless, timely diagnosis and subsequent treatment are needed to avoid its sequelae. The purposes of this article are to review the history and nature of forearm compartment syndrome, review the pertinent anatomy, describe the potential etiologies, and review the pathophysiology, treatment strategies, and potential outcomes and complications.

HISTORY

Volkmann is credited with the original description of compartment syndrome in 1881.[12] He attributed the end result of myonecrosis to splints that led to diminished arterial inflow, which ultimately led to muscle ischemia and cell death. Hildebrand, in 1890, is credited with first using the term *Volkmann contracture*, described later. The first myofascial release for impending compartment syndrome was described in 1890 by Bardenhauer.[13] Sixty years after the first description of compartment syndrome by Volkmann, in 1940, Griffiths described arterial injury and reflex spasm of the collateral vessels as the source of muscle ischemia. He also minimized the role of tight dressings and splints as the cause of diminished arterial inflow.[13,14] Also described in Griffiths' original work are what is now known as the 5 Ps of compartment syndrome: pain, pallor, paresthesias, paralysis, and eventually pulselessness.

Since the 1970s, understanding of the basic science and pathophysiology of compartment syndrome has considerably increased. Rorabeck and Clarke[15] recognized that there was not only damage to muscles due to compartment syndrome but also that associated nerves traversing the compartment also had the potential to be damaged. They showed that if compartmental release was performed within 4 hours of onset that nerve conduction velocity always returned to normal regardless of the amount of pressure applied or the length of time the pressure was applied. If the release was performed after 12 hours, however, then nerve conduction velocity did not return to normal at any pressure or time condition, demonstrating the possibility of irreversible nerve damage if compartment syndrome is not diagnosed and treated early.

Experimental studies by Whitesides and colleagues[16] focused on muscle damage and introduced the concept of measuring tissue pressures to identify the need for fasciotomy in suspected compartment syndrome. They showed that after 4 hours of muscle ischemia less than 5% of muscle cells were damaged; however, if ischemia time was prolonged to 8 hours then nearly 100% of muscles were damaged.[14] Whitesides and colleagues[16] described inadequate perfusion of muscle cells when the tissue pressure within a closed compartment rose to within 10 to 30 mm Hg of the diastolic blood pressure.

ETIOLOGY

There are a variety of causes of forearm compartment syndrome reported in the literature. Fractures of the forearm and fractures of the distal radius are the most common causes of forearm compartment syndrome (**Fig. 1**).[1] There is no difference in reported compartment syndrome occurrences between open and closed fractures of the forearm.[17] Other causes, such as burns, crush injuries, penetrating trauma, constrictive dressings or casts, infections, bleeding disorders, extravasation of drugs or intravenous fluids, reperfusion injury, and arterial injury, have all been reported.[18] The wide variety of reported causes necessitates a thorough history and physical examination by the treating surgeon, which can be particularly difficult in polytraumatized patients with distracting injuries or patients who are obtunded. The obtunded patient with a potential forearm compartment syndrome poses a particularly difficult challenge. These patients may also include the "found down" population, who come in obtunded with no history; therefore, the onset and duration of symptoms is most often unknown unless a friend or family member accompanies them.

PATHOPHYSIOLOGY

Compartment syndrome is defined as a condition in which a closed osseofascial compartment's pressure increases to such an extent that there is a compromise of the microcirculation to that compartment leading to tissue damage.[19] Tissue perfusion is proportional to the difference between capillary perfusion pressure and the interstitial fluid pressure. The normal resting pressure in the adult

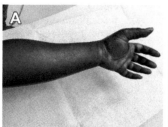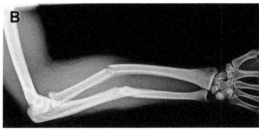

Fig. 1. (*A*) Note a swollen forearm with the swelling extending into the fingers. (*B*) Radiograph notes a fracture of the midshaft of the radius and ulna. Fractures are the most common cause of compartment syndrome of the forearm. (*Courtesy of* [*A*] Katharine Criner, MD, Philadelphia, PA.)

forearm has been reported to be 0 mm Hg to 8 mm Hg.[14] Tissue fascia is avascular and nonelastic; therefore, it is resistant to acute stretching and creates a fixed space housing the muscles of the forearm.[20] As the pressure in the forearm increases due to injury or external forces, the venous pressure also rises, which results in a decrease in the arteriovenous pressure gradient. The increasing venous pressure leads to increased interstitial fluid pressure ultimately reducing the local perfusion of tissues. The result is tissue edema, a reduction in lymphatic drainage, and ultimately more tissue edema and rising tissue pressure that result in a repeating cycle of events, or positive feedback loop, that only ceases if decompression of the compartment is performed.[21] The end result of this cycle is tissue ischemia and cell death (**Fig. 2**).

ANATOMY

The forearm is the most common site of compartment syndrome in the upper extremity.[1,14] There are 4 compartments in the forearm and a thorough understanding of this complex anatomy is necessary for proper treatment of compartment syndrome. The 4 compartments include the volar compartment, both superficial and deep; the dorsal compartment; and the mobile wad. Burkhart and colleagues[22] describe up to 10 compartments of the forearm that are not strictly separated from each other but rather aligned by interconnections. For the purpose of this review, however, the focus is on the 4 functional compartments of the forearm.

The interosseous membrane of the radius and ulna divides the forearm into the volar and dorsal compartments. The deep volar compartment is most susceptible to ischemic and compressive injury due to fascial boundaries that prevent expansion of the muscle bellies during injury. The deep volar compartment lies immediately volar to the interosseous membrane. This compartment

includes the flexor pollicus longus (FPL) and the flexor digitorum profundus (FDP). The pronator quadratus is also included in the deep volar compartment; however, this muscle is located more distal within the forearm and some investigators consider it a separate compartment because elevated tissue pressures can affect it independently from the other forearm muscles.[23] Immediately volar to the deep volar compartment are the muscles of the superficial volar compartment, which include the pronator teres, palmaris longus, flexor digitorum superficialis (FDS), flexor carpi radialis (FCR), and flexor carpi ulnaris (FCU). The lacertus fibrosus (bicipital aponeurosis) is a fascial extension of the distal extent of the biceps tendon that inserts into the pronator fascia and can also be a source of compression around the elbow and routinely should be released during decompressive fasciotomy.

Within the volar compartments run the median nerve proper, the anterior interosseous nerve (AIN), and the ulnar nerve. Due to its deeper course in the forearm between the FDS and FDP, the median nerve is the most commonly injured nerve with forearm compartment syndrome. It is often found encased in heavy scar in the setting of Volkmann ischemic contracture.[21] The AIN runs in the floor of the deep volar compartment and innervates the deep flexors. Therefore, the deep compartment can experience devastating consequences of compartment syndrome, including both irreversible muscle and nerve damage. The ulnar nerve run is bounded in the midforearm by the FDS, the FCU, and the FDP. It is often subject to injury with a compartment syndrome but not necessarily to the extent the median nerve is.

The dorsal compartment lies dorsal to the interosseous membrane and houses the finger extensors: extensor digitorum communis, extensor digiti minimi, extensor carpi ulnaris, abductor pollicis longus, extensor pollicis longus, extensor pollicis brevis, extensor indicis proprius, and the

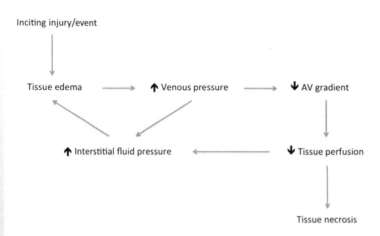

Fig. 2. The cycle of ischemia and tissue death brought on by compartment pressure exceeding arterial perfusion pressure. AV, arteriovenous.

supinator muscle. The anconeus has also been described as a potential independent compartment.[14] The dorsal compartment is not as frequently injured in forearm compartment syndrome compared with the deep flexor muscles. The posterior interosseous nerve (PIN) is the continuation of the deep branch of the radial nerve and runs on the floor of the dorsal compartment to innervate all the muscles on the dorsal and radial aspect of the forearm except the anconeus, brachioradialis, and extensor carpi radialis longus (ECRL).

Finally, the mobile wad is the fourth main compartment described in the forearm and includes the brachioradialis, extensor carpi radialis longus, and extensor carpi radialis brevis (ERCB). This compartment begins at the origins of these muscles on the lateral aspect of the humerus and extends distally to the wrist. These muscles are the most infrequently injured in acute compartment syndrome due to their superficial location and because they are easily decompressed. The radial nerve proper runs in the floor of the mobile wad to innervate the brachioradialis, ECRL, and the anconeus. The ECRB has variable innervation from either the radial nerve proper or the PIN. The radial nerve proper and its deep branch, the PIN, are infrequently damaged in forearm compartment syndrome due to their relatively superficial location.

DIAGNOSIS

The diagnosis of compartment syndrome of the forearm is usually on the basis of clinical signs and symptoms. It requires a high index of suspicion given the wide variety of injuries that have been attributed to the development of forearm compartment syndrome. Classically, the hallmarks have been the 5 Ps: pain out of proportion, pallor, paresthesias, paralysis, and pulselessness. A sixth symptom, pain with passive stretching, is now also included as part of the diagnostic signs. Pain out of proportion and pain with passive stretching of the fingers are considered the first and most sensitive signs of compartment syndrome in an awake patient. In contrast, pulselessness is a late-stage or even end-stage symptom and compartment syndrome has usually been present for some time before pulses are lost.[21] The other clinical signs of compartment syndrome have a poor predictive value because previous studies have shown them to have a low sensitivity but high specificity for diagnosis. Also, it is not uncommon to have the diagnosis made after a period of time of observation because the signs and symptoms generally evolve over a period of hours after initial presentation.[24] If 3 of the clinical signs and symptoms are present, then it has been reported that there is greater than 90% probability that a compartment syndrome is present.[25] The authors' recommendation, however, is that further objective data be obtained or empiric fasciotomy be performed before all the clinical signs and symptoms are present because irreversible damage has likely occurred if the patient gets to the late stages of the disease process. It is also critical for the treating surgeon to assess the hand because separate hand compartment releases may also be needed if they are swollen and tense.

Patients typically present with a tense and swollen forearm that may or may not be in the setting of a fracture. If there is an open fracture of the forearm present, the clinician should not dismiss the possibility of forearm compartment syndrome in thinking that the hematoma will extravasate from the open wound, allowing decompression of the compartment.[2] In delayed presentations, it is possible to also have skin manifestations, including blistering.[21] An important step after initial clinical assessment is to remove any bandages or splints that may be causing external compression on the forearm. Any fractures that are displaced should also be provisionally reduced, which can alleviate increased pressure in the forearm by restoring soft tissue relationships. If, after clinical assessment and provisional fracture reduction, the diagnosis remains equivocal, then objective data should be obtained, particularly in obtunded or unresponsive patients and in the pediatric population.

There are several methods that have been developed to measure compartmental pressures, including arterial line transducer systems, slit catheters, and self-contained measuring systems.[24] The normal resting pressure in an adult forearm has been reported to be 8 mm Hg to 9 mm Hg.[21] Currently, the accepted guideline for the diagnosis of compartment syndrome is a pressure measurement that is within 30 mm Hg of the diastolic blood pressure. Some clinicians accept the diagnosis of compartment syndrome, however, if the absolute pressure in the compartment is greater than 30 mm Hg. When using a compartmental pressure monitoring device, it is imperative that all 4 compartments in the forearm be measured to ensure that the diagnosis is not missed because it is possible for one or all of the compartments to be elevated in the setting of an injury. If both the clinical and objective data support the diagnosis of forearm compartment syndrome, then emergent fasciotomy is indicated.

Weick and colleagues[26] examined new alternative methods to obtain objective data for the diagnosis of compartment syndrome. They used an animal model to take direct measurements of tissue oxygenation and found that the partial pressure of oxygen was decreased in limbs with induced compartment syndrome and then subsequently rose when the limb was decompressed with fasciotomy. This method has yet to be tested in humans but is an area of future research that could aid in better diagnostic methods.

MANAGEMENT

Forearm compartment syndrome is a surgical emergency and must be recognized and treated early with surgical decompression and fasciotomy to avoid irreversible sequelae, including muscle and nerve damage. Although there have been case reports in the literature describing nonoperative treatment, this is not recommended in the setting of a true compartment syndrome, and any patient treated successfully with nonoperative treatment likely never had a true compartment syndrome to begin with. There are a small number of patients, depending on the initial presentation and possible etiology, who can undergo a trial of nonoperative management and observation (ie, removal of tight bandages or splints); however, there should be an extremely low threshold to proceed with compartment pressure measurement or decompression if these patients do not rapidly improve.

The management of forearm compartment syndrome first and foremost requires a high clinical suspicion and rapid delivery to the operating room. Although the compartment syndrome may be biased toward a particular compartment, the authors recommend empiric decompression of all compartments. Classically, surgical decompression of all forearm compartments is accomplished with 2 incisions, 1 on the volar aspect and 1 on the dorsal aspect of the forearm. A pneumatic arm tourniquet should be avoided in the setting of forearm fasciotomy to properly assess postdecompression perfusion.

The volar forearm incision begins proximal and medial to the antecubital fossa and extends distally to the radial forearm in a curvilinear fashion and then curves back to the ulnar forearm at the level of the distal third of the forearm and then back to the midline at the level of the carpal tunnel to aid in carpal tunnel release (**Fig. 3**). This extended curvilinear incision allows for easy decompression of the median nerve in the carpal tunnel and creates a radially based skin flap to allow adequate skin coverage of the median nerve in the volar forearm because the wound is usually large with edematous skin edges. The proximal aspect of the incision allows access to visualization and decompression of the lacertus fibrosus.

Once the skin incision has been made the superficial flexor compartment is assessed and decompressed with a fascial incision from the lacertus fibrosus to the wrist flexion crease. After adequate decompression of the superficial volar compartment, it is imperative that deep volar compartment be inspected and released because the deep flexors are more commonly compromised in the setting of forearm compartment syndrome. It is also important to individually inspect the pronator quadratus because some investigators have opined that this muscle is contained within a separate compartment, as discussed previously.[23] After all volar compartments have been released, the surgeon must carefully inspect muscle tissue perfusion to ensure that adequate blood flow is present. Any necrotic muscle encountered

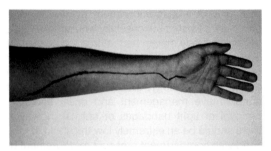

Fig. 3. Volar incision of a forearm compartment release. Note the extensile nature, beginning with a carpal tunnel release distally, an oblique wrist incision crossing the wrist away from the palmar cutaneous nerve, and proximal extension across the elbow medially allowing access to the lacertus fibrosus to facilitate proximal decompression of the median nerve.

at the time of initial decompression should be sharply débrided.

There are additional volar surgical approaches that have been described in the literature. Ronel and colleagues[23] conducted a literature review of the surgical approaches to the volar forearm (the ulnar approach described by McConnell, the central approach described by Thompson, and the radial approach described by Henry). They found that all 3 approaches allowed easy access for decompression of the superficial volar compartment. They found that an ulnar approach to the deep volar compartment created the least amount of iatrogenic injury to the superficial musculature but all approaches allowed adequate decompression of the deep volar compartment. Although the authors use the incision and approach described in **Fig. 3**, any approach is valid if adequate visualization and release of the volar compartment are achieved.

The dorsal compartment and mobile wad are decompressed with a single midline incision beginning at the level of the lateral epicondyle and extending to the distal radioulnar joint in line with Lister tubercle. Often the muscles of the dorsal forearm can be contained within fascial septae that need to be individually decompressed.[14] The same principles of perfusion assessment apply to the dorsal compartment and mobile wad.

Some investigators have advocated that complete forearm decompression can be accomplished with a single volar incision. Ojike and colleagues[27] performed a cadaveric study in which compartment pressure measurements were taken both before and after surgical decompression with a single volar incision in induced compartment syndrome in cadaver forearms. They found that pressure measurements in all 3 compartments returned to near baseline

10 minutes after decompression. If the treating surgeon chooses to proceed with a single volar incision for forearm arm decompression, the dorsal compartment must be closely monitored postoperatively to avoid damage to the wrist extensors from an inadequate volarly based decompression of the dorsal compartment.[21]

Once adequate decompression of all forearm compartments has been achieved, the wounds must be appropriately managed. The surgical incisions are best left open to avoid the recreation of compressive forces on the compartments with early attempted closure. Moreover, primary closure is typically not possible acutely due to excessive tissue edema. Typically, tissue edema increase within the first 24 hours to 48 hours after fasciotomy due to reperfusion. Some surgeons apply retention sutures to the wounds to avoid skin edge retraction.[1,21] The wounds are dressed with sterile wet-to-dry dressings or a negative pressure wound therapy (NPWT) device can be applied. The patient is returned to the operating room every 48 hours to 72 hours after initial fasciotomy to examine and irrigate the wounds and débride any additional muscle necrosis as it declares itself. The wounds can be closed primarily in a delayed fashion once edema has subsided but often split-thickness skin grafts are necessary for soft tissue coverage. Healing by secondary intention has been abandoned due to increased risk of infection, prolonged hospital course, increased incidence of muscle necrosis and sepsis, and delay in rehabilitation.[28] The use of NPWT has been shown to reduce the need for skin grafting, result in shorter hospital stays, and decrease the rate of nosocomial infections.[1,29] The use of NPWT also has the added benefits of draining excess fluid from the forearm, which ultimately results in decreased pressure and edema and contributes to improved blood flow to the area.[29] NPWT can be used in conjunction with other methods of wound closure, including delayed primary closure and skin grafting.

Many efforts have been made to determine the best method for fasciotomy wound closure. Kalyani and colleagues[30] conducted a systematic review and found that for patients who underwent fasciotomy for forearm compartment syndrome 39% were able to undergo delayed primary closure and 61% had to undergo postfasciotomy skin grafting. Rogers and colleagues[31] compared skin grafting to delayed linear closure of fasciotomy wounds and found that those patients who underwent delayed linear closure had shorter hospital stays and were more satisfied with their scars postoperatively compared with those patients treated with skin grafting. The skin graft cohort underwent fewer operations, however, during their hospital course. Wilkin and colleagues[29] found that the use of NPWT for compartment syndrome wounds in a pig model resulted in reduced skeletal muscle fiber regeneration. The results of this study, however, have not been evaluated in a human population and the benefits of NPWT, as previously described, must be weighed against the possible risks, including wound infection and sepsis.

OUTCOMES AND COMPLICATIONS

The outcomes and complications of forearm compartment syndrome are dependent on a variety of factors, including injury severity, ischemia time, and associated comorbidities. Time from diagnosis to fasciotomy, however, seems the most important factor that contributes to outcomes with the general recommendation for patients to undergo decompression within 6 hours to 24 hours from the time of diagnosis.[1]

In a recent systematic review of forearm compartment syndrome, the overall complication rate was found to be 42%, with neurologic deficit reported the most common complication.[30] Other reported complications include contractures (9.3%), gangrene (2.3%), Volkmann ischemic contracture (2.3%), crush syndrome (4.7%), and complex regional pain syndrome (2.3%). Duckworth and colleagues[32] reported a complication rate of 32% in their cohort of acute forearm compartment syndrome, with neurologic deficit also the most common complication (18%). They reported that a delay in the time to decompression was predictive of long-term complications. If patients underwent fasciotomy after 6 hours of presentation, then they were significantly more likely to develop complications, including neurologic deficit, contracture, delayed fracture union, muscle necrosis, and tethering of skin graft to tendon limiting motion.

Many times the actual onset of compartment syndrome is unknown when a patient arrives at the hospital; so even when rapid intervention is appropriately provided patients can still develop residual dysfunction. One of the most devastating complications is Volkmann ischemic contracture, which results from muscle necrosis caused by irreversible tissue ischemia. Tsuge[33] classified the resulting contracture as mild, moderate, or severe. The mild type includes mild contracture of the FDP, no contracture of the extensor tendons, and no to minimal neurologic findings. The moderate type includes contracture of the FDP and FPL with variable findings of the FDS, FCU, and FCR. There are usually no extensor complications;

however, the moderate type typically has neurologic symptoms in the median nerve distribution. Finally, the severe type involves contractures of all the flexor muscles in the volar forearm, variable findings of the extensor muscles, and severe neurologic problems in the both the medial and ulnar distributions, and they can have joint contractures, bone deformities, and skin scarring.

The main goal of treatment of Volkmann ischemic contracture is restoration of function; however, it should be established with the patient that normal function of the arm and hand should not be expected.[1,21] Once all the involved muscles are identified, treatment begins with aggressive débridement of the nonfunctioning muscle along with neurolysis of the median and ulnar nerves and tenolysis of any tendons that have become scarred down. Tendon lengthening has not had good results in clinical practice and has been shown associated with recurrence of contracture.[34] Tendon transfers can be performed in patients with mild or moderate contracture and usually involve transfer of an extensor tendon when they are not involved. Ultee and Hovius[34] reported substantial improvement in function in patients who underwent free vascularized muscle transplantation, but this treatment should be reserved for those patients with the severe form of Volkmann ischemic contracture.[21,34] Unfortunately this procedure can involve donor site morbidity because most commonly a free gracilis transfer is used and it requires microsurgical expertise.

SUMMARY

Because forearm compartment syndrome can have devastating sequelae, early diagnosis and decompressive fasciotomy is essential for the patient. Given the large variety of causes that have been reported in the literature, careful history and physical examination by the treating surgeon are paramount. When a patient is unable to give a history or proper examination is not possible due distracting injuries or the patient being obtunded, then objective clinical data in the form of compartment pressure measurements should be obtained. If the clinical scenario warrants it, however, then it is not unreasonable to progress to empiric decompressive fasciotomies. Understanding of the pathophysiology and etiology of compartment syndrome has improved greatly in the past 40 years but the treatments of the potential disabilities that can result from compartment syndrome remain suboptimal and are not without complications themselves. This should be an area of continued research in the future.

REFERENCES

1. Prasarn ML, Ouellette EA. Acute compartment syndrome of the upper extremity. J Am Acad Orthop Surg 2011;19(1):49–58.
2. Elliot KG, Johnstone AJ. Diagnosing acute compartment syndrome. J Bone Joint Surg Br 2003;85(5):625–32.
3. Sayar U, Ozer T, Mataraci I. Forearm compartment syndrome caused by reperfusion injury. Case Rep Vasc Med 2014;2014:931410.
4. Omori S, Miyake J, Hamada K, et al. Compartment syndrome of the arm caused by transcatheter angiography or angioplasty. Orthopedics 2013;36(1):e121–5.
5. Chinn M, Colella MR. Prehospital dextrose extravasation causing forearm compartment syndrome: a case report. Prehosp Emerg Care 2017;21(1):79–82.
6. Alexander CM, Ramsmeyer M, Beatty JS. Missed extravasation injury from the peripheral infusion of norepinephrine resulting in forearm compartment syndrome and amputation. Am Surg 2016;82(7):162–3.
7. Pare JR, Moore CL. Intravenous infiltration resulting in compartment syndrome: a systematic review. J Patient Saf 2015. [Epub ahead of print].
8. Halpern AA, Mochizuki R, Long CE. Compartment syndrome of the forearm following radial artery puncture in a patient treated with anticoagulants. J Bone Joint Surg Am 1978;60(8):1136–7.
9. Funk L, Grover D, de Silva H. Compartment syndrome of the hand following intra-arterial injection of heroin. J Hand Surg Br 1999;24(3):366–7.
10. Cohen J, Bush S. Case report: compartment syndrome after a suspected black widow spider bite. Ann Emerg Med 2005;45(4):414–6.
11. Ilyas AM, Wisbeck JM, Shaffer GW, et al. Upper extremity compartment syndrome secondary to acquired factor VIII inhibitor: a case report. J Bone Joint Surg Am 2005;87(7):1606–8.
12. Volkmann R. Die ischaemischen muskellahmungen und kontrakturen. Centralbl Chir 1881;8:801–3.
13. Green DP, Wolfe SW. Green's operative hand surgery. Philadelphia: Elsevier/Churchill Livingstone; 2017.
14. Leversedge FJ, Moore TJ, Peterson BC, et al. Compartment syndrome of the upper extremity. J Hand Surg Am 2011;36(3):544–59.
15. Rorabeck CH, Clarke KM. The pathophysiology of the anterior tibial compartment syndrome: an experimental investigation. J Trauma 1978;18(5):299–304.
16. Whitesides TE, Haney TC, Morimoto K, et al. Tissue pressure measurements as a determinant for the need of fasciotomy. Clin Orthop Relat Res 1975;(113):43–51.
17. Janzing HM. Epidemiology, etiology, pathophysiology and diagnosis of the acute compartment syndrome of the extremity. Eur J Trauma Emerg Surg 2007;33(6):576–83.
18. Donaldson J, Haddad B, Khan WS. The pathophysiology, diagnosis, and current management of acute compartment syndrome. Open Orthop J 2014;8:185–93.
19. Raza H, Mahapatra A. Acute compartment syndrome in orthopedics: causes, diagnosis, and management. Adv Orthop 2015;2015:543412.
20. Fry WR, Wade MD, Smith RS, et al. Extremity compartment syndrome and fasciotomy: a review. Eur J Trauma Emerg Surg 2013;39(6):561–7.
21. Friedrich JB, Shin AY. Management of forearm compartment syndrome. Hand Clin 2007;23(2):245–54.
22. Burkhart KJ, Mueller LP, Prommersberger KJ, et al. Acute compartment syndrome of the upper extremity. Eur J Trauma Emerg Surg 2007;33(6):584–8.
23. Ronel DN, Mtui E, Nolan WB. Forearm compartment syndrome: anatomical analysis of surgical approaches to the deep space. Plast Reconstr Surg 2004;114(3):697–705.
24. von Keudell AG, Weaver MJ, Appleton PT, et al. Diagnosis and treatment of acute extremity compartment syndrome. Lancet 2015;386(10000):1299–310.
25. McQueen MM, Duckworth AD. The diagnosis of acute compartment syndrome: a review. Eur J Trauma Emerg Surg 2014;40(5):521–8.
26. Weick JW, Kang H, Lee L. Direct measurement of tissue oxygenation as a method of diagnosis of acute compartment syndrome. J Orthop Trauma 2016;30(11):585–91.
27. Ojike NI, Alla SR, Battista CT, et al. A single volar incision will decompress all three forearm compartments: a cadaver study. Injury 2012;43(11):1949–52.
28. Kakagia D. How to close a limb fasciotomy wound: an overview of current techniques. Int J Low Extrem Wounds 2015;14(3):268–76.
29. Wilkin G, Khogali S, Garbedian S, et al. Negative-pressure wound therapy after fasciotomy reduces muscle-fiber regeneration in a pig model. J Bone Joint Surg Am 2014;96(16):1378–85.
30. Kalyani BS, Fisher BE, Roberts CS, et al. Compartment syndrome of the forearm: a systematic review. J Hand Surg Am 2011;36(3):535–43.
31. Rogers GF, Maclellan RA, Liu AS, et al. Extremity fasciotomy wound closure: comparison of skin grafting to staged linear closure. J Plast Reconstr Aesthet Surg 2013;66(3):e90–1.
32. Duckworth AD, Mitchell SE, Molyneux SG, et al. Acute compartment syndrome of the forearm. J Bone Joint Surg Am 2012;94(10):e63.
33. Tsuge K. Treatment of established Volkmann's contracture. J Bone Joint Surg Am 1975;57(7):925–9.
34. Ultee J, Hovius SE. Functional results after treatment of Volkmann's ischemic contracture: a long-term followup study. Clin Orthop Relat Res 2005;(431):42–9.

Traumatic Wounds of the Upper Extremity
Coverage Strategies

Muhammad Mustehsan Bashir, FCPS (Plastic Surgery), FCPS (Surgery)[a],
Muhammad Sohail, FCPS (Plastic Surgery), FCPS (Surgery)[b],*,
Hussan Birkhez Shami, MBBS[c]

KEYWORDS

• Soft tissue coverage • Upper limb reconstruction • Flap • Trauma

KEY POINTS

• Inadequate management of traumatic wounds of the upper extremity may lead to amputation or permanent disability and can be a major cause of psychological distress.
• Soft tissue coverage is required to salvage traumatized limbs and restore adequate function and form.
• An optimal coverage should be stable, durable, and able to withstand heavy demands of work; should allow free joint mobility; and should have an aesthetically acceptable appearance.
• Both autologous tissue and dermal skin substitutes can be used for coverage. Autologous coverage ranges from simple skin grafts to complex free flaps.

INTRODUCTION

Traumatic wounds of the upper extremity often result from serious and devastating injuries involving multiple components, including skin, bone, tendon, and neurovascular structures, which may threaten limb survival or impair limb function. Complex injuries commonly result from road traffic, workplace, or domestic accidents; assaults; and burns. Other mechanisms of injury include sharp, crush, avulsion, high-pressure, gunshot, explosion, thermal, chemical, electrical, or combined injuries.

Inadequate management can lead to amputation or permanent disability and is a major cause of psychological distress. Skin coverage is often required to salvage a limb with restoration of adequate function and form. An optimal coverage should be stable, durable, and able to withstand heavy demands of work; should allow free joint mobility; and should have aesthetically acceptable appearance.[1–3]

This article provides a summary of commonly used soft tissue reconstructive strategies for traumatic wounds of the upper extremity.

INITIAL EVALUATION AND MANAGEMENT IN EMERGENCY ROOM

On initial contact in the emergency room (ER), assess vitals and stability based on Advanced Cardiac Life Support and Advanced Trauma Life Support guidelines. In stable patients with no life-threatening and limb-threatening injuries, begin

Disclosure: All authors have approved the article and its submission. No funding in cash or kind was involved.
Conflicts of Interest: The authors declare that they have no conflicts of interest.
[a] Department of Plastic, Reconstructive Surgery and Burn Unit, King Edward Medical University, Mayo Hospital, House No 327-block-H DHA, Phase 5, Lahore, Pakistan; [b] Department of Plastic, Reconstructive Surgery and Burn Unit, King Edward Medical University, Mayo Hospital, 86A Habibullah Road, Garhi Shahu, Lahore, Pakistan; [c] Department of Plastic, Reconstructive Surgery and Burn Unit, King Edward Medical University, Mayo Hospital, Lahore, Pakistan
* Corresponding author.
E-mail addresses: drsohail72@gmail.com; drsohail@kemu.edu.pk

Hand Clin 34 (2018) 61–74
https://doi.org/10.1016/j.hcl.2017.09.007
0749-0712/18/© 2017 Elsevier Inc. All rights reserved.

with a history focusing on clinical characteristics, comorbidities, profession, duration, mechanism, and severity of injury along with hand dominance, and associated injuries. Also note the status of tetanus prophylaxis, smoking, allergies, and time of last meal. Initial physical examination should be focused to determine suitability of the limb and injured parts for potential salvage, replantation, or use as spare parts. In particular, attention should be spent on the wound, focusing on extent and type of injury, contamination, extent of the defect, and neurovascular status of the injured limb. If grossly contaminated, wound cultures can be sent. Plain radiographs with the appropriate views should also be obtained to confirm or rule out skeletal injuries.[1–4]

URGENT REEVALUATION AND SURGICAL MANAGEMENT OF WOUNDS

In patients who can tolerate a surgical procedure, reevaluation should be performed in sterile conditions, under general anesthesia, with tourniquet control. It should be focused to achieve the following goals[1,4,5]:

- Removal of contamination (eg, foreign bodies mud, grease, oil)
- Identification and grading the severity of the injury
- Control of bleeding
- Layer-by-layer debridement of severely devitalized tissues
- Stabilization of bone and joints
- Restoration of circulation by microsurgical direct repair or grafting
- In selective and suitable condition, primary repair and reconstruction of nerves and tendons
- Soft tissue closure/coverage (**Fig. 1**)

TIMING OF WOUND CLOSURE/COVERAGE

- Primary wound closure with or without flap and with or without primary repair or reconstruction of other structures (tendon and nerves) is performed within 12 to 24 hours.[5,6]
- Delayed primary flap coverage with delayed reconstruction is done within 2 to 7 days.
- Secondary flap coverage with delayed reconstruction is best done after 7 days.

PRIMARY SOFT TISSUE WOUND CLOSURE/ COVERAGE

Primary closure should be planned for patients who are able to tolerate prolonged surgery and whose wounds are clean.

VACUUM-ASSISTED CLOSURE THERAPY

Vacuum-assisted closure (VAC) therapy is a simple method for both temporary wound coverage and optimization of the wound bed. The device works by application of controlled negative pressure to the wound in cyclical fashion. The negative pressure removes blood or serous fluid, thus decreasing edema and dead space, reducing bacterial count and potential infection, and increasing microperfusion and neovascularization of the wound bed. In many cases, application of VAC therapy can avoid the use of flaps for coverage of the wound[7,8](**Fig. 2**A,B).

STRATEGIES FOR SKIN AND SOFT TISSUE COVERAGE

Options for coverage are autologous tissue and dermal skin substitutes.[9] Choice of reconstructive technique depends on age of patient, nature and duration of trauma, wound characteristics, and condition of surrounding tissues. Exposed vital structures and need for secondary procedures also affect the selection of the optimum coverage technique.

Skin Grafts

Skin grafting is the most commonly performed procedure for coverage of defects that are not suitable for primary closure. A vascularized and healthy recipient bed is required for graft survival. VAC is a useful tool to help prepare a recipient bed for a graft. Relative contraindications to a primary skin graft include exposed tendon, nerves, bones, blood vessels, and joints. Choice of graft (full or split thickness) depends on condition and duration of wound, amount of dermis required, and location of defect. Full-thickness skin grafts (FTSGs) are generally more durable but do not stretch, result in larger donor site defects, and can be less sensate. Split-thickness skin grafting may be less durable but can stretch, are ultimately more sensate, do not result in donor site coverage needs, and can be more versatile. For example, meshing a split-thickness skin graft can avoid collection of blood or serum under the graft and can provide greater coverage area. However, a meshed graft gives a pebbled appearance. For a graft to take well, whether full or split thickness, it should be applied directly on a clean and vascularized recipient bed with a layered compression nonadherent dressing and immobilized against stress or shear[10] (**Fig. 2**).

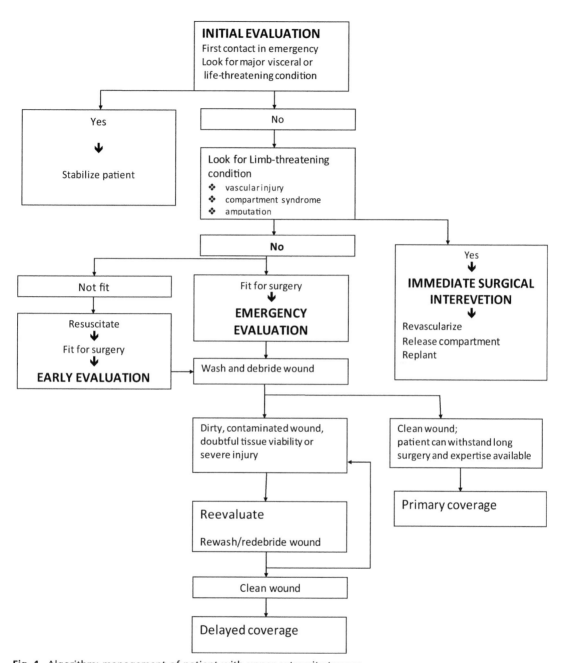

Fig. 1. Algorithm: management of patient with upper extremity trauma.

Synthetic Skin Substitutes

Dermal skin substitutes can provide skin coverage even when deep structures such as bone, tendon, and neurovascular structures are exposed on a healthy vascular bed. The most commonly used dermal skin substitute material currently is Integra (Integra LifeSciences, Plainsboro, NJ), which is a scaffold of bovine collagen mixed with chondroitin sulfate and covered with a semipermeable silicone membrane. Once the scaffold incorporates into a wound bed, usually after 21 days, the silicone membrane is removed and a split-thickness skin graft is applied. Some dermal substitutes, like Allo-Derm, can be applied with immediate skin grafting performed over them. Skin substitutes provide an acceptable aesthetic appearance with favorable functional outcome. On many occasions, use of dermal substitutes has obviated the use of flaps

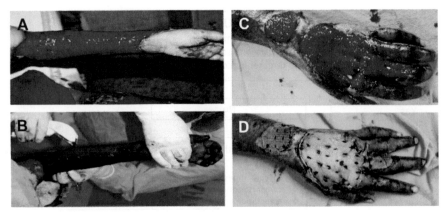

Fig. 2. Case 1. (*A*) Preoperative view of wound left elbow and forearm (after VAC therapy) with healthy granulation tissue without exposure of any vital structure. (*B*) Postoperative view after split-skin grafting. (*C*) Preoperative view of wounds on dorsum of left hand and elbow with healthy granulation tissue. (*D*) Postoperative view after split-skin graft.

because they can be used to cover small areas of exposed tendons, bone, and nerves in an otherwise healthy vascular bed[11] (**Fig. 3**).

Flaps

Flaps are traditionally indicated for coverage of wounds with exposed tendon, nerves, bones, blood vessels, and joints (**Table 1**). Hand defects are unique and any reconstructive tissue needs to facilitate free tendon and joint mobility, and therefore should be strong enough to withstand daily heavy work forces while also maintaining sensibility of the hand.[4,12,13] Common flap options for the hand include local advancement or rotation flaps, regional flaps, and free flaps.[14]

Local advancement flaps

Atasoy V-Y volar advancement flap Atasoy V-Y volar advancement flap is used for coverage of dorsal fingertip defects. The flap is marked over the volar skin of distal phalanx as a V with tip at the distal interphalangeal crease. The flap is

elevated above the flexor sheath and advanced distally to cover the defect with V-Y donor site closure. It provides sensate coverage and avoids midline scar[15,16] **Fig. 4**B.

Kutler bilateral V-Y advancement flap Two lateral V-shaped flaps are used to provide sensibility and padding for transverse or dorsal fingertip defects. Flaps are raised from the sides of the injured finger as triangles with the tip at the distal interphalangeal joint and the base at the defect's border. Particular attention should be paid to protecting terminal branches of the neurovascular bundles lying in the lateral pulp tissue of the flap. The flap is elevated above the flexor tendon sheath, advanced distally, and stitched in the midline with V-Y donor site closure[17,18] (**Fig. 4**A).

Moberg advancement flap This robust flap is based on perforating branches of ulnar and radial digital arteries of the thumb. It consists of the entire volar surface of the injured thumb, which is advanced to cover volar tip defects. Taking both

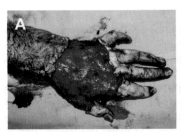
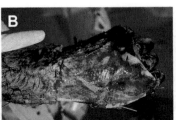
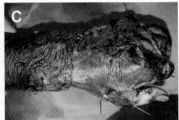

Fig. 3. (*A*) Preoperative view of wound over dorsum of left hand. (*B*) Dermal skin substitute (AlloDerm) applied to resurface the defect. (*C*) View after split-skin grafting over dermal substitute.

Table 1
Options for coverage of traumatic wounds of the upper limb

	Hand	Forearm	Elbow	Arm
Local flaps	Kutler Atasoy Reverse homodigital Moberg advancement	Transposition Rotation Rhomboid Propeller	Transposition Rotation	Transposition Rotation Rhomboid
Regional flaps	Cross-finger Littler neurovascular FDMA Reverse RFF Reverse UFF Reverse PIA	For volar surface PIA UFF For dorsal surface RFF UFF	Proximally based RFF/UFF/PIA Distally based lateral arm flap	Lateral arm Medial arm
Distant flaps	Groin Abdominal	Groin Abdominal	Thoracoepigastric LD	LD/TDAP Parascapular
Free flaps	Contralateral radial forearm Latissimus dorsi Anterolateral thigh flap Scapular and parascapular Lateral arm flap			

Abbreviations: FDMA, first dorsal metacarpal artery flap; LD, latissimus dorsi flap; PIA, posterior interosseous artery flap; RFF, radial forearm free flap; TDAP, thoracodorsal artery perforator flap; UFF, ulnar forearm flap.

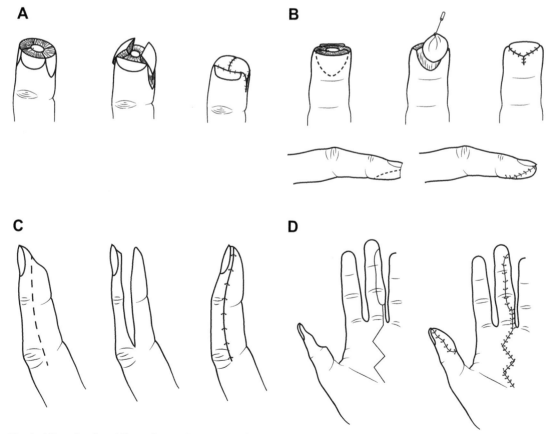

Fig. 4. (*A*) Kutler flap: bilateral V-Y advancement flaps for fingertip injuries. (*B*) Atasoy flap: a single V-Y advancement flap for fingertip injuries. (*C*) Moberg flap: the advancement flap for thumb injuries. (*D*) Littler flap: defect of thumb distal portion, which can be resurfaced with a Littler flap tunneled through the palm before the flap donor site is grafted.

digital arteries does not hamper the blood supply of the thumb because this is also perfused by princeps pollicis artery. The flap is raised superficial to the flexor tendon sheath. Some limited flexion of the thumb interphalangeal joint is often required for tension-free closure; however, this may lead to joint stiffness and/or contracture. The Moberg flap may be converted to an islanded flap and may also be extended over the thenar eminence in a V fashion with V-Y closure of the donor site[19] (**Fig. 4**C).

Regional flaps

Littler neurovascular island flap The Littler flap involves the transfer of sensate glabrous tissue from the ulnar border of the ring or long finger for coverage of defects of the distal tip of the same digit, thumb, or adjacent digits. The flap is based on the digital neurovascular bundle and designed over the volar lateral aspect of the digit. The flap is dissected preserving the paratenon but incorporating the neurovascular bundle. The neurovascular bundle of the other side of the ipsilateral digit should be protected to maintain vascularity from the donor finger. The flap is advanced distally for coverage of same-finger defects with V-Y donor closure. For resurfacing the thumb and adjacent fingers, the pedicle is dissected up to the proximal palmar crease and is transferred directly or tunneled onto the thumb defect. The donor site is covered with FTSG or planter skin. The flap has a disadvantage of some sensory deficit over the donor finger[20,21] (**Fig. 4**D).

Cross-finger flap A cross-finger flap is a reliable flap for coverage of volar digital defects. It uses tissue from an adjacent finger based on branches of the dorsal digital artery. The flap is designed over the dorsal aspect of the middle or proximal phalanx and raised off the extensor tendon paratenon along the lateral border away from the recipient finger. The flap is then flipped and sutured to the recipient finger's volar defect margins. The donor site is then grafted with an FTSG from the ipsilateral proximal medial arm.

In contrast, a reverse cross-finger flap is used to cover defects on the dorsal aspect of digits. First, a very thin skin flap is raised based on the opposing side of the designed flap. Then the designed flap is raised, consisting of subcutaneous tissue only. The flap is flipped over and its dermal surface is applied to the dorsal defect of the adjacent recipient finger. The donor site is then covered with an FTSG.

Either flap can be depedicled at 2 weeks. Disadvantages of this technique are the need for 2-stage procedures, inferior aesthetic appearance with skin color mismatch, and joint stiffness from prolonged immobilization[22,23] (**Fig. 5**).

First dorsal metacarpal artery or kite flap This flap is perfused by the first dorsal metacarpal artery (FDMA) and provides sensate tissue for coverage of the defects of the thumb, first web space, and palmar aspect of the index finger. The flap uses dorsal skin of the proximal phalanx of the index finger. The flap is elevated off the extensor tendon paratenon. A subcutaneous pedicle of the same width as that of the flap is elevated in a subfascial plane, including the FDMA, superficial veins, and dorsal superficial branches of the radial nerve. The donor site is covered with an FTSG. The flap may also be raised on reverse flow based on palmar perforators at the metacarpal neck or further distally on communication between the dorsal metacarpal artery and the dorsal phalangeal branches. The donor defect is covered with an FTSG. A reverse-flow flap is less reliable than a proximally based flap[24,25] (**Fig. 6**).

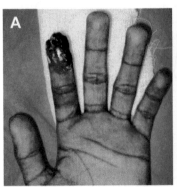
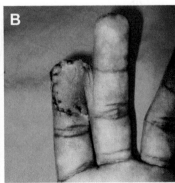
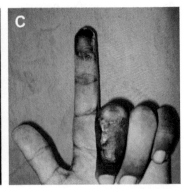

Fig. 5. (*A*) Preoperative view of wound over the volar aspect of left index finger involving the distal phalanx with exposed tendon. (*B*) Cross-finger flap from the dorsal aspect of the middle phalanx of the middle finger has been used to resurface the defect. (*C*) Postoperative view after division and insetting of the flap and healed skin graft over flap donor site.

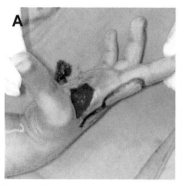
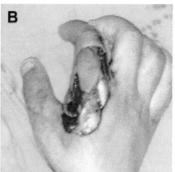
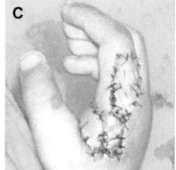

Fig. 6. (*A*) Preoperative view of defect first web space of right hand. (*B*) FDMA flap has been raised. (*C*) Postoperative view after flap insetting. The flap donor site has been skin grafted.

Reverse homodigital islanded flap This flap uses skin of the proximal part of the same digit based on reverse flow in the digital artery. It provides sensate coverage to fingertip defects with excellent color and texture match. Further advantages include single-stage coverage with primary closure of the donor defect[26] (**Fig. 7**).

Radial forearm flap A distally based radial forearm flap is perfused on retrograde flow through the deep palmar arch and associated venae comitantes. It is easy to harvest and provides thin and hairless skin at the expense of the radial artery. It can be used for coverage of the defects of wrist, palm, dorsum of the hand, proximal fingers, and thumb. A preoperative Allen test is performed to determine the patency of the palmar arch and ensure the vascularity of the hand based on the ulnar artery alone. Venous drainage occurs by crossover and bypassing valves. The skin island is designed on the volar aspect of the proximal forearm centered on the flap axis. The flap is raised either subfascially or suprafascially, incorporating the radial artery and associated venae comitantes, and preserving a layer

of paratenon and sensory branches of the radial nerve. The donor site is covered with an FTSG. The flap may be modified as an adipofascial, fascial-only, or even osteofasciocutaneous flap. Donor site scarring is a common drawback, but the flap is otherwise robust and versatile[27] (**Figs. 8** and **9**).

Reverse posterior interosseous artery flap This flap provides pliable and thin coverage for defects of the dorsal aspect of the hand, wrist, thumb, and first web space. The flap is perfused by retrograde flow through the anastomotic branches of the posterior interosseous artery (PIA) and the anterior interosseous artery (AIA) and does not sacrifice any of the 2 major arteries to the hand. The flap is centered on the middle third of the axis drawn on the dorsal aspect of the forearm from the lateral epicondyle of the humerus to the distal radioulnar joint. The flap is raised subfascially from proximal to distal, incorporating the PIA and cutaneous perforators until the anastomotic branch of the AIA is reached. Closure of the donor defect up to 6 cm can be achieved primarily. The posterior interosseous nerve should be protected

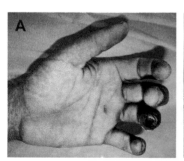
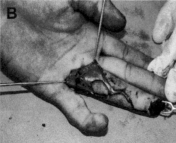
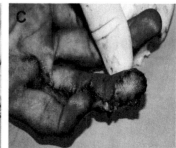

Fig. 7. (*A*) Preoperative view of a defect involving the tip of the left ring finger with exposed bone. (*B*) A homodigital flap based on the ulnar side of the digit has been raised. (*C*) Postoperative view of the flap after insetting.

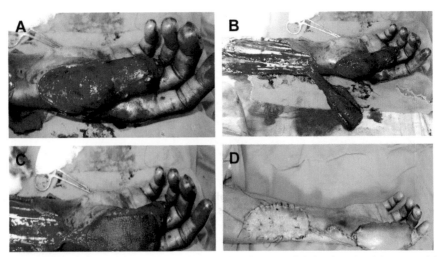

Fig. 8. (*A*) Preoperative view showing wound involving the dorsum of right thumb with exposed bone. (*B*) A distally based islanded radial forearm flap has been raised to resurface the defect. (*C*) View showing the flap's reach. (*D*) Postoperative view showing the flap insetting and a skin-grafted flap donor site.

because it runs close to vascular pedicle on its radial side. The constraints of using this flap are the limited availability of tissue and tedious dissection[28] (**Fig. 10**).

Distally based ulnar artery forearm flap This thin flap is reliable and can be used to cover defects of the wrist, palm, dorsum of hand, and proximal fingers. The flap is based on reverse flow of the ulnar artery through the deep palmar arch. Because it sacrifices ulnar arterial supply to the hand, the flap may be modified as a perforator flap. The flap is centered on an axis drawn from the medial epicondyle of the humerus to the lateral edge of the pisiform. The ulnar nerve should be protected from injury during dissection. The flap is transposed to cover the defect. For large donor defects, an FTSG is applied[29,30] (**Fig. 11**).

Becker dorsoulnar flap This flap is based on a perforating branch of the ulnar artery. It has the advantages of providing thin, hairless skin

without sacrificing any major vessel. The flap is designed as a reverse U over a line drawn from the medial epicondyle proximally to the ulnar neck distally with a pivot point 2 to 3 cm proximal to the pisiform. The flap is elevated either suprafascially or subfascially. Branches of the medial cutaneous nerve of the forearm are scarified during flap elevation. However, dorsal branches of the ulnar nerve should be preserved. Small donor defects can be closed primarily[31] (**Fig. 12**).

Distant flaps
Groin flap The flap is based on the superficial circumflex iliac artery (SCIA). It is designed as an ellipse centered on an axis from the femoral vessels medially to the anterior-superior iliac spine laterally, 2 to 3 cm below the inguinal ligament. The flap may extend 5 to 10 cm around the trunk, and a width of up to 10 to 12 cm may be harvested with primary closure of the donor site. Dissection is performed in the suprafascial plane until the

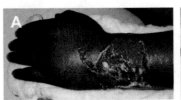
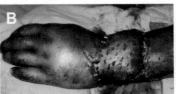
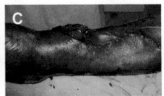

Fig. 9. (*A*) Preoperative view showing defect over the extensor aspect of the distal forearm with exposed bone and tendons. (*B*) The distally based adipofascial radial forearm free flap covered with split-thickness skin graft. (*C*) Preoperative view showing the donor site, which has been closed primarily.

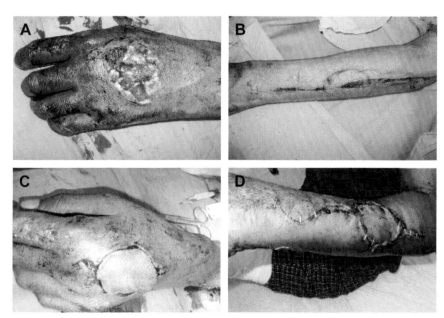

Fig. 10. (*A*) Preoperative view of the wound over the extensor surface of hand. (*B*) Distally based PIA flap is marked. (*C*) The defect is resurfaced with flap. (*D*) Postoperative grafted donor site.

sartorius is reached, at which point dissection is extended deep to the fascia to include the SCIA because it runs deep at this level. The dissection is ultimately continued to the medial border of the sartorius. The recipient hand is placed in the appropriate position and the defect is covered with the flap. The flap can later be depedicled at 3 weeks[32,33] (**Fig. 13**).

Abdominal flap The flap is based medially on the periumbilical perforators or inferiorly on the superficial inferior epigastric artery. Abdominal flaps are very reliable flaps and provide abundant tissue for coverage of large defects. Flaps based on periumbilical perforators can safely be extended to the midaxillary line. The flap is elevated superficial to muscle fascia. The flap can be depedicled at

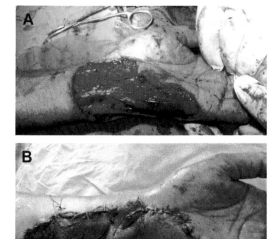

Fig. 11. (*A*) Preoperative view of wound involving the hypothenar region of left hand with exposed tendons. (*B*) Postoperative view after wound coverage with ulnar artery flap.

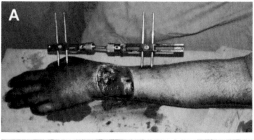

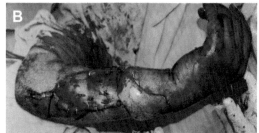

Fig. 12. (*A*) Preoperative view of wound involving left wrist surface with exposed tendons. (*B*) Postoperative view after Becker dorsoulnar flap coverage. The donor defect was skin grafted.

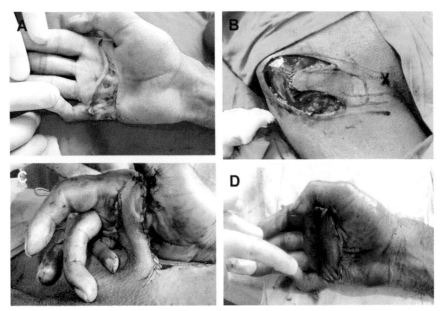

Fig. 13. (*A*) Preoperative view of wound to right hand with exposed tendons. (*B*) Groin flap has been marked and raised. (*C*) Flap sutured to cover the defect. (*D*) Postoperative view after division and insetting of the flap.

3 weeks. The required 2 stages and the bulk of the tissue are this flap's 2 major drawbacks[34] (**Fig. 14**).

Free flaps

Free tissue transfer for upper extremity wound coverage is preferred when other options are not available or the defect is not amenable to coverage by other options. Free flaps provide freedom of movement of tissue for coverage in a single stage with acceptable donor site morbidity. However, the requirement for microvascular expertise and availability of facilities for microvascular free-tissue transfer may be limiting factors.[35] Factors determining the selection of free flaps are given in **Box 1**.

Optimal timing of free flaps for soft tissue coverage of upper extremity traumatic wounds is still debatable. Many reports have mentioned

that delaying free-tissue transfer for 6 to 8 days decreases the failure rate. However, many others advocate coverage within 72 hours because it reduces the risk of edema and infection and helps earlier recovery of the patient, which decreases patient suffering and hospital length of stay and also helps in earlier rehabilitation. However, some studies have found that there is no effect of timing on the outcomes of free flaps.[36] A brief description of the most commonly used free flaps for soft tissue coverage of upper limb is presented here.

Radial forearm free flap This robust flap is a preferred choice for coverage of the upper extremity because of its many advantages, such as thinness of skin, long pedicle with large caliber of vessels for anastomosis, and the multitude of

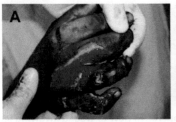
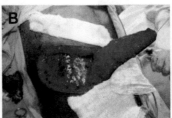
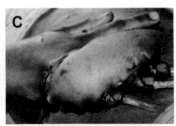

Fig. 14. (*A*) Preoperative view of wound to right hand involving dorsal aspect of the ulnar 3 digits with exposed tendon. (*B*) Abdominal flap based on the right paraumbilical perforators has been raised exposing the underlying abdominal muscle. (*C*) Postoperative view of the same patient with flap covering all the 3 digits.

structures that can be harvested with it. Single or multiple skin islands can also be harvested. The flap is elevated on a proximal vascular pedicle. Inclusion of cutaneous vein in large flaps helps in avoiding venous congestion. The flap may be harvested as an adipocutaneous, fascial-only, osteofasciocutaneous, myocutaneous, tendinocutaneous, or vascularized nerve flap (superficial radial nerve), or as a flow-through flap. The main disadvantage is the conspicuous donor scar, especially in women, but this can be decreased with suprafascial flap harvesting and full-thickness grafting of the donor defect.[27,37,38]

Anterolateral thigh flap The anterolateral thigh flap is based on the descending branch of the lateral circumflex femoral artery. It provides a large skin paddle, fascia, and vastus lateralis muscle with minimal donor site morbidity. It has sufficiently long pedicle with good diameter for anastomosis. A skin island is designed on a line drawn from the anterior-superior iliac spine to the lateral border of the patella. Reliable perforators are located roughly midway down this line. Dissection begins medially and is continued laterally until the skin perforators are identified. The main pedicle is identified and dissected to its origin. Closure of donor defects less than or equal to 7 cm in width can be achieved primarily. Variation in perforator anatomy, transfer of hairy skin, and excess bulk are the main disadvantages[39,40] (**Fig. 15**).

Scapular and parascapular free flap Both flaps are based on the circumflex scapular artery (CSA), a branch of the subscapular artery. Its advantages include provision of a large, hairless skin paddle and well-hidden scar. The scapular flap is

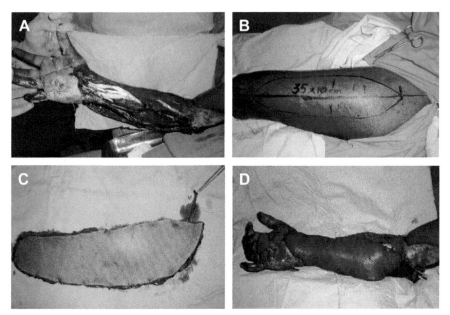

Fig. 15. (*A*) Preoperative view of the wound involving the right hand and forearm after debridement with exposed tendons. (*B*) Marked left anterolateral thigh flap. (*C*) The flap has been divided and is ready to be transferred. (*D*) Postoperative view after flap inset and anastomosis.

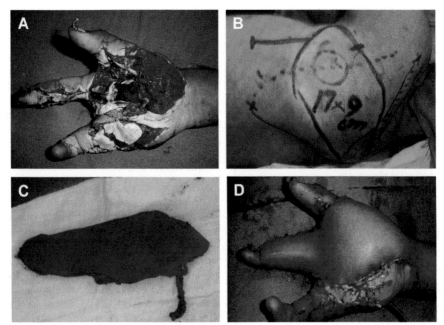

Fig. 16. (*A*) Preoperative view of traumatic wound to right hand with amputated middle and ring finger and exposed tendons. (*B*) Marked parascapular flap. (*C*) The flap has been divided and is ready to be transferred. (*D*) Postoperative view after flap inset and anastomosis.

designed transversely along the spine of scapula and the parascapular flap is sited obliquely along the lateral border of the scapula, and they are based on transverse and descending branches of the CSA respectively. The flap is dissected in the subfascial plane (**Fig. 16**). The flap pedicle length is 4 to 6 cm at its origin from the subscapular artery, which can be increased with inclusion of the artery. To provide larger amounts of tissue for reconstruction, either or both flaps may be harvested in combination with the latissimus dorsi and serratus anterior muscle flaps on a single common subscapular pedicle as a chimeric flap (**Fig. 17**). Having to reposition the patient from a prone or lateral position for flap harvesting is the primary limitation and inconvenience of this flap.[38,41]

Free latissimus dorsi flap The latissimus dorsi flap is very reliable and this is the largest single muscle for coverage of large upper extremity defects. This versatile flap is based on the thoracodorsal artery, which is a continuation of the subscapular artery. Loss of muscle function at the donor site is compensated for by the action of the teres major and pectoralis major muscles. Easy harvesting and a long pedicle (8–11 cm) with large-diameter vessels makes this an ideal flap. The flap is also versatile and may be modified as segmental, neurotized (functioning) muscle, and can be musculocutaneous or skin only. A cutaneous paddle is usually designed as an ellipse and can be oriented horizontally, transversely, or obliquely. Donor

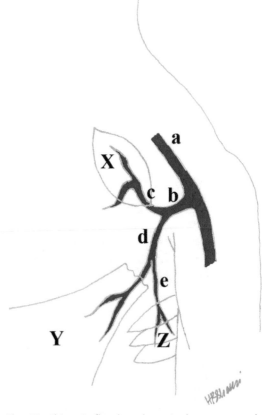

Fig. 17. Chimeric flap based on single common subscapular system. a, axillary artery; b, subscapular artery; c, circumflex scapular artery; d, thoracodorsal artery; e, branch to serratus; X, parascapular flap; Y, latissimus dorsi flap; Z, serratus anterior muscle flap.

defects are closed primarily. Seroma formation at donor site is a common sequela. The need for intraoperative patient repositioning and a long scar on the back are the main limitations of this flap.[38]

Lateral arm free flap The lateral arm free flap is based on the posterior radial collateral artery and its septocutaneous perforators. This flap has the advantage of harvesting from the ipsilateral arm without sacrificing any major vessel. The main disadvantages are short pedicle length with small arterial diameter for anastomosis, limited skin availability for coverage, forearm dysesthesia, and visible donor scar. The flap may be raised simply as a fascial flap to decrease donor site morbidity. During elevation of the flap, the radial nerve running beside the pedicle must be protected from injury. The flap may be modified as a sensate flap (with inclusion of the posterior cutaneous nerve of the arm), an osteocutaneous flap, or as a flow-through flap.[38]

SUMMARY

Timely soft tissue coverage with autologous tissue or dermal skin substitutes helps in limb salvage and restoration of aesthetic and functional outcomes. Local tissue is considered ideal for smaller defects; however, larger defects require regional or free flaps. Free flaps provide easy movement of tissue in a single stage compared with regional flaps; however; they require microvascular expertise and facilities.

ACKNOWLEDGMENTS

The authors acknowledge Dr Falak Sher Malik, Assistant Professor (Orthoplastic Surgeon, Department of Plastic, Reconstructive and Hand Surgery, GTTH/LMDC Lahore), for contributing **Figs. 16** and **17** for this article.

REFERENCES

1. Alphonsus CK. Principles in the management of a mangled hand. Indian J Plast Surg 2011;44(2): 219–26.
2. Griffin M, Hindocha S, Malahias M, et al. Flap decisions and options in soft tissue coverage of the upper limb. Open Orthop J 2014;8:409–14.
3. Langer V. Management of major limb injuries. ScientificWorldJournal 2014;2014:640430.
4. Latifi R, ElHennawy H, ElMenyar A, et al. The therapeutic challenges of degloving soft-tissue injuries. J Emerg Trauma Shock 2014;7(3):228–32.
5. Cheema T. Principles of treating complex hand injuries. In: Cheema T, editor. Complex injuries of the hand. London: JP Medical; 2014. p. 51–74.
6. Hansen SL, Lang P, Sbitany H. Soft tissue reconstruction of the upper extremity. In: Thorne CH, Chung KC, Gosain AK, et al, editors. Grab and Smith's plastic surgery. 7th edition. Philadelphia: Lippincott William & Wilkins; 2014. p. 737–49.
7. Kneser U, Leffler M, Bach AD, et al. Vacuum assisted closure (V.A.C.) therapy is an essential tool for treatment of complex defect injuries of the upper extremity. Zentralbl Chir 2006;131(1):S7–12.
8. Lambert KV, Hayes P, McCarthy M. Vacuum assisted closure: a review of development and current applications. Eur J Vasc Endovasc Surg 2005;29(3):219–26.
9. Ng ZY, Salgado CJ, Moran SL, et al. Soft tissue coverage of the mangled upper extremity. Semin Plast Surg 2015;29(1):48–54.
10. Thorne CH. Techniques and principles in plastic surgery. In: Thorne CH, Chung KC, Gosain AK, et al, editors. Grab and Smith's plastic surgery. 7th edition. Philadelphia: Lippincott William & Wilkins; 2014. p. 1–12.
11. Ellis CV, Kulber DA. Acellular dermal matrices in hand reconstruction. Plast Reconstr Surg 2012; 130(Suppl. 2):256S–69S.
12. Huang JM, Wiedrich TA. Local hand flaps. J Am Soc Surg Hand 2001;1(1):25–44.
13. Eberlin KR, Chang J, Curtin CM, et al. Soft-tissue coverage of the hand: a case-based approach. Plast Reconstr Surg 2014 Jan;133(1):91–101.
14. Biswas D, Wysocki RW, Fernandez JJ, et al. Local and regional flaps for hand coverage. J Hand Surg Am 2014;39(5):992–1004.
15. Thoma A, Vartija LK. Making the V-Y advancement flap safer in fingertip amputations. Can J Plast Surg 2010;18(4):e47–9.
16. Atasoy E, Ioakimidis E, Kasdan ML, et al. Reconstruction of the amputated finger tip with a triangular volar flap. A new surgical procedure. J Bone Joint Surg Am 1970;52(5):921–6.
17. Sungur N, Kankaya Y, Yıldız K, et al. Bilateral V-Y rotation advancement flap for fingertip amputations. Hand (N Y) 2012;7(1):79–85.
18. Kutler W. A new method for finger tip amputation. J Am Med Assoc 1947;133(1):29.
19. Macht SD, Watson HK. The Moberg volar advancement flap for digital reconstruction. J Hand Surg Am 1980;5(4):372–6.
20. Adani R. Heterodigital flaps for severe pulp defects. BMC Proc 2015;9(3):A60.
21. Yıldırım AR, iğde M, Tapan M, et al. Littler flap: a reliable option in soft tissue defects of different fingers. Cumhuriyet Med J 2016;38(4):332–9.
22. Koch H, Kielnhofer A, Hubmer M, et al. Donor site morbidity in cross-finger flaps. Br J Plast Surg 2005;58(8):1131–5.

23. Rajappa S, Prashanth T. Cross finger flap cover for fingertip injuries. Int J Res Orthop 2017;3(2):164–7.

24. Prabhu M, Powar R, Sulhyan SR. FDMA flap: a versatile technique to reconstruct the thumb. Int J Pharm Med & Bio Sc 2013;2(4):8–14.

25. Makkar RM, Naemm W, Naeem J, et al. The innervated 1st dorsal metacarpal artery island flap for reconstruction of post traumatic thumb defects. Egypt J Plast Reconstr Surg 2012;36(2):147–52.

26. Momeni A, Zajonc H, Kalash Z, et al. Reconstruction of distal phalangeal injuries with the reverse homodigital island flap. Injury 2008;39(12):1460–3.

27. Jones NF, Jarrahy R, Kaufman MR. Pedicled and free radial forearm flaps for reconstruction of the elbow, wrist, and hand. Plast Reconstr Surg 2008; 121(3):887–98.

28. Cavadas PC, Ibañez J, Landin L, et al. Use of the reversed posterior interosseous flap in staged reconstruction of mutilating hand injuries before toe transfers. Plast Reconstr Surg 2008;122(6): 1823–6.

29. Ignatiadis IA, Giannoulis FS, Mavrogenis AF, et al. Ulnar and radial artery based perforator adipofascial flaps. EEXOT 2008;59(2):101–8.

30. Grobbelaar AO, Harrison DH. The distally based ulnar artery island flap in hand reconstruction. J Hand Surg Br 1997;22(2):204–11.

31. Becker C, Gilbert A. The ulnar flap – description and applications. Eur J Plast Surg 1988;11(2):79–82.

32. Goertz O, Kapalschinski N, Daigeler A, et al. The effectiveness of pedicled groin flaps in the treatment of hand defects: results of 49 patients. J Hand Surg Am 2012;37(10):2088–94.

33. Jokuszies A, Niederbichler AD, Hirsch N, et al. The pedicled groin flap for defect closure of the hand. Oper Orthop Traumatol 2010;22(4):440–51 [in German].

34. Ali A, Farg M, Safe K. Reconstruction of hand and forearm defects by abdominal thin skin flaps. Egypt J Plast Reconstr Surg 2007;31(2):181–5.

35. Horta R, Silva P, Costa-Ferreira A, et al. Microsurgical soft-tissue hand reconstruction: an algorithm for selection of the best procedure. J Hand Microsurg 2011;3(2):73–7.

36. Harrison BL, Lakhiani C, Lee MR, et al. Timing of traumatic upper extremity free flap reconstruction: a systematic review and progress report. Plast Reconstr Surg 2013;132:591.

37. Kruavit A, Visuthikosol V, Punyahotra N, et al. Radial forearm free flap. Thai J Surg 2004;25(1):7–22.

38. Antohi N, Stingu C, Stan V. The use of free flap transfer in upper extremity reconstruction. TMJ 2005; 55(1):27–35.

39. Abdelkader R, Hossam El Mahdy, Khairalla TN, et al. The antero-lateral thigh flap in coverage of extensive post traumatic upper limb defects. Surg Sci 2016;7: 309–15.

40. Hsu CC, Lin YT, Lin CH, et al. Immediate emergency free anterolateral thigh flap transfer for the mutilated upper extremity. Plast Reconstr Surg 2009;123:1739.

41. Hashmi PM. Free scapular flap for reconstruction of upper extremity defects. J Coll Physicians Surg Pak 2004;14(8):485–8.

Elbow Fractures with Instability
Evaluation and Treatment Strategies

Neal C. Chen, MD

KEYWORDS

- Elbow • Fracture • Dislocation • Instability • ORIF

KEY POINTS

- Initial management of elbow fracture dislocations include evaluation of the shoulder and wrist, neurovascular examination, and assessment of the skin for open wounds. If grossly dislocated, a preliminary reduction is recommended.
- Elbow fractures with ulnohumeral instability tend to occur in 5 general patterns: (1) terrible triad, (2) varus posteromedial rotatory instability, (3) olecranon fracture dislocation, (4) radial head fracture with ulnohumeral dislocation, and (5) lateral column fracture of the distal humerus with ulnohumeral dislocation.
- Loose or incompetent repair of the collaterals and/or not repairing small coronoid fractures are common causes of residual instability after repair.
- There is no consensus regarding the management of the ulnar nerve; however, the nerve should be managed thoughtfully.
- A stiff, congruent elbow is preferable to an unstable elbow. If intraoperative instability after repair persists, external fixation, internal hinge, or internal static fixation are recommended.

INTRODUCTION

The treatment of elbow fractures with ulnohumeral instability is in evolution. In the past, unstable elbow fractures were considered as variations of the same injury, but more recently, computed tomography (CT) scans have helped us recognize that there are distinct groups of fracture patterns. These patterns help predict what structures are injured and guide treatment.

Improvements in radial head arthroplasty, soft tissue repair, and spanning implant technologies are also important in better outcomes. Midterm results are substantially improved than in the past; however, long-term outcomes are uncertain.

INITIAL MANAGEMENT

Apart from the standard trauma assessment, the management of an elbow fracture dislocation should include evaluation of the shoulder and wrist and a neurovascular examination. Skin integrity is assessed and open wounds are treated promptly with local wound care.

Radiographs of the shoulder, elbow, and wrist are obtained. Gentle traction views are obtained if the patient is reasonably comfortable. CT scans with 3-dimensional reconstructions are useful to understand the fracture.

If the ulnohumeral joint or radiocapitellar joint is grossly dislocated, reduction is recommended; but in some cases, the ulnohumeral joint will remain subluxated because of the fracture pattern and multiple attempts at reduction may not be beneficial. In either case, the limb is splinted until definitive treatment.

UNDERSTANDING THE INJURY

Radiographs and CT scans can be used to make a judgment about the overall stability of the elbow or

Hand and Upper Extremity Service, Department of Orthopaedic Surgery, Massachusetts General Hospital, Harvard Medical School, 55 Fruit Street, Boston, MA 20114, USA
E-mail address: nchen1@partners.org

Hand Clin 34 (2018) 75–83
https://doi.org/10.1016/j.hcl.2017.09.008
0749-0712/18/© 2017 Elsevier Inc. All rights reserved.

hand.theclinics.com

forearm as well as the stability of the fractured bones.

Fractures of the proximal radius or ulna can involve instability of the ulnohumeral joint, proximal radioulnar joint (Monteggia fracture), or forearm (Essex-Lopresti).

Elbow fractures with ulnohumeral instability tend to occur in general patterns: (1) terrible triad, (2) varus posteromedial rotatory instability (VPMRI), (3) olecranon fracture dislocation (OFD), (4) radial head fracture with ulnohumeral dislocation, and (5) lateral column fracture of the distal humerus with ulnohumeral dislocation. A terrible triad consists of a fracture of the radial head, fracture involving the olecranon tip, and rupture of the lateral collateral ligament (LCL). VPMRI consists of a fracture of the anteromedial coronoid facet and rupture of the LCL. OFDs consist of a fracture of the olecranon with dislocation/subluxation of the intact forearm relative to the distal humerus. This is usually accompanied by a radial head fracture.

It is important to distinguish OFD from a Monteggia fracture. Monteggia described this fracture predating the discovery of x-rays, and the term Monteggia fracture or Monteggia variant has been used broadly to describe almost any ulna fracture with instability of the radiocapitellar articulation. Our practice has found it helpful to strictly define Monteggia fracture as a fracture of the proximal ulna with proximal radioulnar joint instability to improve our understanding and communication about elbow injuries. There is overlap between OFD and Monteggia fractures when there is a large degree of proximal ulna comminution.

An Essex-Lopresti lesion involves dissociation of the ulna from the radius. Usually, there is a fracture of the radial head proximally and a disruption of the distal radioulnar joint distally. The distal injury may also involve a distal radius fracture or intercarpal injury such as a perilunate dislocation.

ELEMENTS OF FRACTURE-INSTABILITY PATTERNS
Coronoid

The shape and size of the coronoid fracture can help distinguish among the terrible triad, VPMRI, and OFD instability patterns.[1] O'Driscoll and colleagues[1] classified coronoid fractures into 3 types: tip, anteromedial facet, and base fractures. In general, coronoid tip fractures are associated with terrible triad injuries, coronoid anteromedial facet fracture with VPMRI injuries, and a coronoid base fracture is associated with OFD injuries.[2] In patients with a chronically subluxated elbow, the coronoid may erode and the instability of the

elbow may become more difficult to address to restore stability.

Radial Head

Fractures of the radial head in the setting of ulnohumeral instability are generally more complex than isolated radial head or neck fractures. Duckworth and colleagues[3] describe elbow injuries involving the radial head occurring in a "stable" or "unstable" setting.[3] Stable injuries usually have an intact periosteum and are unlikely to displace, whereas unstable injuries occur with large soft tissue disruptions and gross mechanical instability of the elbow.

The area of the radial head that is injured can be larger than that identified on radiographs or even CT scan. When partial articular fractures occur in the unstable elbow, there is often comminution at the fracture margin.[4] In addition, partial articular fractures tend to occur in the anterolateral portion of the radial head, an area important for biomechanical stability.[5]

Collateral Ligament Injury

Both collateral ligaments are injured in simple acute elbow dislocations (dislocations without fracture). In an unstable elbow fracture dislocation, the LCL is frequently avulsed from its origin on the lateral epicondyle. The medial collateral ligament (MCL) is likely injured in most cases, but there is some debate whether proximal avulsion or midsubstance injury is more frequent.[6–8]

In comminuted OFDs, the distal attachment site of the LCL (cristae supinatoris) or the MCL (sublime tubercle) may be fractured from the shaft of the ulna. In these injuries, the proximal origin of the ligaments is usually intact.

SURGICAL PLANNING

Timing of surgery depends on associated injuries, the health of the soft tissue envelope, and availability of resources/implants. Surgery before 2 weeks is preferred, but if a delay is necessary, it is better to optimize resources and have complete preparations rather than perform surgery earlier. Patients who undergo surgery after approximately 2 weeks may benefit from additional stabilization using an external fixator, internal hinge, or pinning the joint to help protect the repaired structures. Outcomes are inferior when definitive treatment occurs after approximately 6 weeks because of soft tissue, bone, and cartilage changes.[9]

Patients may be positioned supine with a bump over the chest or an arm holder, lateral, or prone. If a "push-pull" technique or temporary external fixator is anticipated to reduce a comminuted proximal ulna fracture, supine positioning with an arm holder may be preferable. A c-arm can be brought in from the contralateral side. A sterile tourniquet is preferred. A thoughtful approach toward the sequence of repair of different structures is important. For example, removal of the radial head allows access to the coronoid. This allows the surgeon to avoid a second medial approach in many cases. Another example is if an axis pin is being considered, this should be placed before repairing the LCL and extensor mass.

APPROACHES
Incision

A straight posterior incision or combined medial/lateral incisions may be used. If parallel incisions are used, a general rule of thumb is to have a 1:4 ratio of the distance between incisions and the length of the incision. If possible, it is preferred to minimize undermining the skin bridge between the incisions to preserve skin perforators.

Lateral

There is usually a rent through the common extensor and an avulsion of the LCL. This can be developed proximally and distally. The posterior interosseous nerve crosses the radial neck approximately 3 to 4 cm distal to the radiocapitellar joint and is usually the limit of the distal dissection.[10] If further dissection is needed to expose the proximal radius, the superficial head of the supinator can be split to find the nerve. If a radial head arthroplasty is planned, the radial head can be excised to access the coronoid.

An alternative approach to the proximal radius is to elevate the entire musculature off the lateral ulna (Boyd-Thompson approach). This decreases the risk of injury to the posterior interosseous nerve; however, there is some risk to the distal insertion of the LCL. This approach is particularly useful for fractures of the proximal radius that extend down the shaft or for excision of heterotopic ossification.

Medial

When approaching the medial side of the elbow, the ulnar nerve is identified proximally adjacent to the triceps and released distally through the Osborne ligament and the superficial and deep heads of the flexor carpi ulnaris (FCU). If transposition of the ulnar nerve is planned, approximately 6 to 8 cm of the medial intermuscular septum is excised.

Once freeing the ulnar nerve, the elbow can be approached through 3 methods: (1) using the muscular split along course of the ulnar nerve, (2) splitting the flexor pronator mass anteriorly, or (3) elevating all of the musculature medial to the ulna as one sleeve. To improve proximal access, the flexor pronator mass can be released off the medial epicondyle, similar to a submuscular ulnar nerve transposition. The brachialis can be elevated off the ulna to approach the coronoid anteriorly. The motor branches of the ulnar nerve to the FCU limit distal extension of this approach.

Splitting the flexor pronator mass allows approach to the coronoid as well; however, motor branches from the ulnar nerve to the FCU or to the flexor digitorum profundus to the small finger can also limit distal extension as well. Elevating all the musculature off the elbow is the most extensile distally, but there are risks to injuring the nerve during the deep dissection and it is difficult to reach anterior structures like the coronoid.

Trans-fracture

If the proximal ulna has a transverse fracture and the radial head or coronoid is injured, the injury may be addressed through the existing fracture. When using this approach, it is important to remember the origin and insertion sites of the collateral ligaments and avoid additional injury to these structures during the approach.

TREATMENT FOR SPECIFIC FRACTURE ELEMENTS
Radial Head

If an elbow has dislocated or subluxated and a radial head fracture is present, the radial head is biomechanically compromised. The goal of treatment is either to (1) restore the stability of the elbow so it does not rely on radial head stability or (2) fix or replace the radial head fracture to help restore its biomechanical contribution. The current trend is to repair or replace the radial head because it is not always clear that stability independent of the radial head can be restored. In addition, long-term outcome of Mason 2 fractures where the radial head was repaired demonstrate less arthrosis compared with fractures in which the radial head was excised.[11]

There are various techniques for fracture repair, including screw fixation and plating. Implants should be placed on the nonarticulating portion of the radial head (safe-zone"). This zone correlates to the arc spanning the radial styloid and the Lister tubercle. Hardware outside of this zone may interfere with forearm rotation.

When using screw fixation with oblique screws, it is preferable to use a positioning screw technique rather than a lag or compression screw technique. The goal of positioning screws is to hold the fracture in place, while the goal of lag screws is to compress the fracture. The lag/compression technique can result in malangulation of the radial head fracture.

In fractures with many fragments, one technique is to assemble the fragments of the radial head on the back table and then apply a plate to the fragments proximally and then secure to the neck afterward. This technique can be unforgiving if the plate is malaligned.

If a radial head fracture cannot be repaired solidly, radial head arthroplasty is warranted. There continues to be debate on when a radial head arthroplasty should be used. Ring and colleagues[12] suggest a threshold of 3 radial head fragments or greater. However, most Mason III fractures in this series were treated with plate fixation. Newer evidence suggests that positioning screw fixation of the radial head may be superior to plate fixation with regard to nonunion and failures, and adoption of screw fixation without plating may expand the role of open reduction internal fixation (ORIF) in comminuted radial head fractures.[13]

Radial head arthroplasty can be categorized as unipolar or bipolar. Distally, the prosthesis is fixed or loosely fitting in the proximal radius. All arthroplasty designs demonstrate proximal lucency at midterm follow-up.[14,15] There are some concerns that fixed arthroplasties may be complicated by failure of ingrowth or late loosening.[16,17]

It is important to avoid "overstuffing" or placement of an excessively large prosthesis. A prosthesis may be overstuffed if the elbow has limited range of motion intraoperatively. Suggested radiographic indicators of overstuffing include an asymmetric ulnohumeral joint space and the articular surface of the radial head lying more than 1 mm proximal to the lateral edge of the coronoid.[18,19]

Coronoid

The size of the coronoid fracture dictates options for treatment. For small fragments, the goals of repair are not to fix the actual bony fragments per se, but to provide anterior stability by securing the anterior capsule and soft tissue structures.

In terrible triad injuries, transosseous suture fixation using a lasso provides greater stability and fewer implant failures compared with ORIF or suture anchor fixation.[20]

For larger fragments, the goal of fixation is to secure the fractured bone to create a stable elbow and bony union. This can be achieved using screws with or without a plate. In comminuted fractures, a buttress plate can be applied anteriorly. Occasionally, coronoid fractures cannot be repaired. This situation can occur in patients with chronically unreduced elbows. If the radial head is present, it can be used as a graft to reconstruct the coronoid.[21] If the radial head is not present, other alternatives for graft are the tip of the olecranon, iliac crest autograft, or allograft.[22,23]

Proximal Ulna Fracture

One of the most difficult parts for treatment of proximal ulna fractures is to restore length and alignment. Usually, fracture lines can be visualized to help piece together the fracture anatomically, but in more comminuted fractures, this approach may not be possible. In these situations, use of a push-pull technique or an external fixator can be helpful.

The push-pull technique involves securing the plate on the proximal fracture and then applying the plate distally with a large bone clamp or a Verbrugge clamp. A screw is placed distal to the plate and a laminar spreader or a tensioning device is used to help restore fracture length. Proximal fixation should be secure, as in softer bone, the plate can pull out. The push-pull technique does not provide much rotational control.

In severely comminuted cases in which rotation and length are not clear, application of an external fixator is beneficial. An external fixator pin is placed through a hole in the ulnar plate, the olecranon, through the ulnohumeral joint and into the distal humerus. Smaller caliber external fixator pins are preferred to reduce articular surface injury. A pin is placed in the ulna shaft distal to the anticipated plate length. The external fixator can be manipulated to adjust the rotation and length of the fracture.

Collateral Ligaments

If the proximal origin of the LCL or MCL is avulsed, this can be repaired with suture anchors or transosseous sutures to the epicondyle. Small avulsion fractures of the epicondyle also can be secured using a tension band technique. Sometimes the attachment sites of the MCL or LCL are fractured. They need to be secured to restore stability to the elbow. Sometimes hand fracture plates are better suited to capture these fracture elements.

In chronic cases, the ligaments and soft tissues are attenuated about the elbow. This can be addressed by keeping the elbow stable with adjunct fixation, such as an external fixator, internal hinge, or trans-joint pinning until the soft tissues adjust to the new length/tension.

External fixators can be either static or hinged. When applying an external fixator, the radial nerve can be injured during placement of proximal humeral pins. Making a formal incision can help protect the nerve during pin placement. In the case of a hinged fixator, an axis pin is placed across the distal humerus. The following are tricks to applying an axis pin: (1) place the elbow immediately adjacent to the c-arm receiver, (2) Place soft goods under the elbow to have a stable base, (3) make sure that the elbow is perfectly centered on the image that will make the elbow in line with the x-ray source, (4) place the axis pin and pin driver collinear with the x-ray source. A static fixator or trans-joint pin is generally maintained for 4 weeks. A hinged fixator can be maintained longer.

Internal hinges have been successful in early series.[24,25] They are less bulky and there is no open communication through the skin. Another advantage is malangulation of the humeral axis is less problematic because the hinge is closer to the humerus. In hinged external fixators, the distance of the hinge from the elbow magnifies axis placement error.

ULNAR NERVE

There is no consensus regarding the management of the ulnar nerve; however, there is reasonable evidence that some patients have ulnar nerve dysfunction after elbow fracture dislocations that limit outcomes.[26] If the ulnar nerve is released, the Arcade of Struthers, the proximal brachial fascia, Osborne ligament, and the superficial and deep fascia of the FCU are released. A common guideline is to release the nerve a distance of 6 to 8 cm proximal and distal to the medial epicondyle.

Some surgeons elect to leave the nerve in situ after release, and some surgeons transpose the nerve subcutaneously. If the nerve is transposed subcutaneously, the medial intermuscular septum should be excised a distance of 6 to 8 cm proximal to the medial epicondyle. If an axis pin is to be placed, transposition of the ulnar nerve is generally transposed to prevent injury.

CASE EXAMPLES
Patient 1: Terrible Triad

A 65-year-old woman sustained an elbow injury after a fall from standing height. She underwent manipulative reduction and then operative intervention within approximately 1 week. Radiographs demonstrate a radial head fracture with multiple small bony fragments around the elbow, including a coronoid tip fracture suggestive of a terrible triad injury (**Fig. 1**).

The patient is positioned supine with a hand table and sterile tourniquet. A lateral approach to the elbow allows access to most of the injured structures. There is commonly a soft tissue rent through the lateral structures that is developed proximally.

The radial head is excised. The fragments are retained and used to template the radial head arthroplasty. If the radial head size falls between sizes, a smaller size is selected. The shaft of the proximal radius is prepared. In most systems, the proximal radius is reamed sequentially and then a trial prosthesis is inserted. The trial is removed and the dimensions are recorded.

The coronoid can be visualized once the radial head is excised. A counter incision is made posteriorly on the proximal ulna to expose the dorsal cortex. For transosseous fixation, an anterior cruciate ligament guide or other type of aiming guide is used to drill 2 holes that enter through the dorsal cortex of the ulna and exit in the base of the coronoid fracture. The drill holes should be spaced approximately 1 cm apart on the dorsal cortex. A free end of a #2 or #5-caliber suture is passed through the medial-most hole and then the suture is passed multiple times through the anterior capsule. The needle is removed and then the remaining suture is relayed through the second transosseous hole. The ends of the suture are clamped together.

The actual radial head prosthesis is assembled and inserted. Two suture anchors are placed into the lateral epicondyle. The needles are passed through the lateral soft tissues. At this point, the elbow is placed in a reduced position. The coronoid sutures are tied. The avulsed LCL and lateral soft tissue tissues are tied down without cutting the suture needles. The remaining sutures are then run proximally and distally through the lateral muscle/fascia and then tied.

For rehabilitation, active motion begins at approximately 2 weeks. Gentle stretching can begin at 4 weeks if the elbow is stable. Loading and strengthening begins after the elbow is stable and preferably begins at least after 6 weeks.

Patient 2: Varus Posteromedial Rotatory Instability

A 45-year-old scientist was in a biking accident and sustained a perilunate dislocation and an elbow fracture. The perilunate dislocation was treated acutely and then he was referred for treatment of his elbow fracture. He had an anteromedial coronoid fracture consistent with a VPMRI pattern (**Fig. 2**).

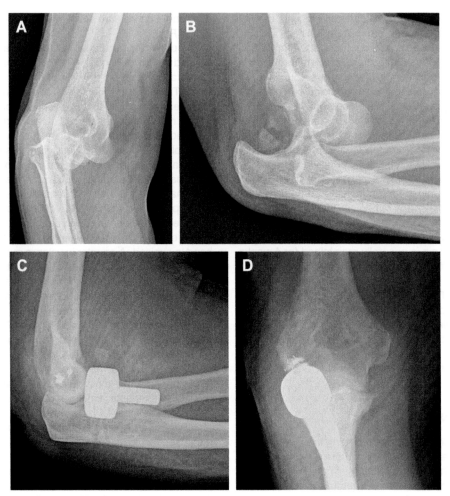

Fig. 1. (*A–D*) Terrible triad treated with radial head arthroplasty, coronoid suture lasso, and suture anchor repair of the LCL. (*Courtesy of* Neal Chen, MD.)

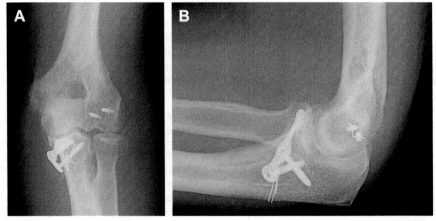

Fig. 2. (*A, B*) VPMRI treated with buttress plating and suture anchor repair of the LCL. (*Courtesy of* Neal Chen, MD.)

The patient is positioned supine with a hand table and sterile tourniquet. A medial approach to the elbow centered over the medial epicondyle is performed. The medial antebrachial cutaneous nerve is identified and the ulnar nerve is released proximally, through the Osborne ligament, and through the FCU. The intermuscular septum is excised and the flexor pronator mass is incised approximately 1 cm distal to the medial epicondyle. The coronoid fracture is identified without detaching the coronoid tip from the soft tissue attachments anteriorly.

A Kirschner wire (k-wire) is driven to prepare for provisional fixation of the coronoid fracture. This can be performed from dorsal to volar using a targeting guide or from volar to dorsal. If going volar to dorsal, 1 or 2 k-wires are placed into the fracture bed and driven through the dorsal cortex until the k-wires are even to the fracture bed. The coronoid is reduced and then the k-wires are advanced into the coronoid fragment.

Once the coronoid is provisionally secured, a plate is applied to the coronoid. Various plates are available. In general, the plate is slightly undercontoured to improve the buttress effect of the plate. A central screw in the plate distal to the fracture is placed, but not completely tightened. The distal end of the plate is pushed anteriorly. This levers the proximal plate to buttress the fracture. A distal screw hole is then secured. Other screw holes are then filled to the surgeon's discretion.

A lateral approach to the elbow is performed. The LCL defect is identified and 1 or 2 suture anchors are placed into the lateral epicondyle. The avulsed LCL is repaired and tied down without cutting off the needles. The remaining suture is run to repair the soft tissue defect distally.

Motion is started approximately 2 weeks after surgery. It is important to avoid varus stress for approximately 6 weeks after the surgery. The elbow experiences varus stress when the arm is held away from the body and the thumb is pointing toward the ceiling. Passive range of motion begins at postoperative week 4. Strengthening begins at approximately 6 weeks.

Patient 3: Olecranon Fracture Dislocation

A 60-year-old woman previously underwent submuscular ulnar nerve transposition wrapped with synthetic fiber in the distant past. She did well for many years, but then fell from standing height and sustained an OFD of the elbow. The radial head/neck is fractured and the olecranon is fractured. The intact forearm is subluxated posterior to the distal humerus and a large coronoid base fracture is noted. The radial head fracture was more complex than appreciated on radiographs and an arthroplasty was performed (**Fig. 3**).

The patient is positioned in lateral position on a beanbag with a sterile tourniquet. A posterior approach to the elbow is performed. The soft tissue attachment to each fracture fragment is preserved. The major proximal olecranon is reflected posteriorly with the triceps attachment to expose the ulnohumeral joint and the radial head. Usually, the forearm can be subluxated posterior relative to the distal humerus to access the radial head and the coronoid.

If needed, the radial head fragments are excised. The fragments are retained and used to template the radial head arthroplasty. If the radial head size falls between sizes, a smaller size is selected. The shaft of the proximal radius is prepared. In most systems, the proximal radius is reamed sequentially and then a trial prosthesis is inserted. The trial is left in place while addressing the coronoid fracture for reference. The actual prosthesis is inserted after the coronoid but before repairing the olecranon.

Major comminuted fragments of the proximal ulna are repaired to the intact shaft. Cannulated screws are helpful to secure the coronoid fragment. Guidewire placement is helpful to anticipate screw entry points. It is important to place screws so they do not interfere with olecranon plate application.

If the length, rotation, and alignment can be reasonably approximated and maintained with a large reduction clamp, the plate is secured provisionally and then the plate is secured.

The elbow is splinted for 2 weeks for wound healing and then active range of motion is initiated. Progression is based on radiographic healing.

PEARLS AND PITFALLS

1. Overlooking small coronoid fractures is one of the more common pitfalls. The fracture may be mistaken for a fragment of the radial head or may be overlooked on radiographs. If there is any doubt, CT scanning can help clarify the injury.
2. Fracture blisters should be allowed to resolve before open surgery even if it takes more than 2 weeks to improve.
3. When approaching the elbow medially, motor branches of the ulnar nerve limit distal dissection. Excessive distal traction can result in palsy

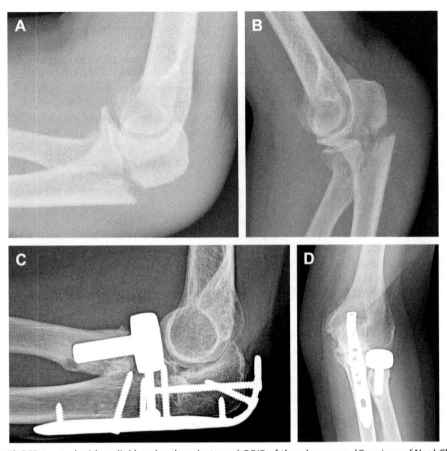

Fig. 3. (*A–D*) OFD treated with radial head arthroplasty and ORIF of the olecranon. (*Courtesy of* Neal Chen, MD.)

of the flexor digitorum profundus of the small finger.

4. If the ulnar nerve is transposed, special attention should be paid to excision of the medial intermuscular septum. The amount of septum excised should be generous. There is usually a vein that perforates the septum approximately 1 cm proximal to the medial epicondyle. I usually excise a width of septum that reaches this perforator medially.

5. Small partial radial head fractures in the setting of the OFD are probably important for stability. Although biomechanical studies have suggested that small fragments can be excised, this option should be used with great caution. It is preferable to fix these small fragments when possible. If not possible, consider radial head arthroplasty.

6. Screw fixation of the coronoid should be performed with some caution. Excessive tightening can cause the coronoid fragment to shatter. In this situation, a buttress plate should be applied.

7. In OFDs, if there is large comminution, special attention should be paid to the attachment sites of the MCL and LCL. These fragments need to be secured to the distal shaft. Hand fracture plates can be helpful to secure these pieces. There is a misconception that the comminuted segment can be bridged, but if these fragments are not secured, the elbow may subluxate or dislocate again.

8. When using the push-pull technique or the external fixation technique, when the radial head aligns with the capitellum on the lateral view and the ulna looks reasonably aligned clinically, this roughly indicates proper alignment and rotation.

9. Overall, a stiff, congruent elbow is preferable to an unstable elbow. If for some reason the elbow cannot be rendered stable by repairing individual elements, reducing the elbow as best as possible and applying a fixator, internal hinge, spanning bridge plate, or pinning the joint is a reasonable salvage option (**Fig. 4**).

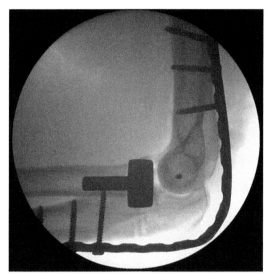

Fig. 4. Temporary spanning bridge plate fixation of an elbow fracture dislocation applied for residual intraoperative instability following repair. (*Courtesy of Asif M. Ilyas, MD, Philadelphia, PA.*)

REFERENCES

1. O'Driscoll SW, Jupiter JB, Cohen MS, et al. Difficult elbow fractures: pearls and pitfalls. Instr Course Lect 2003;52:113–34.
2. Doornberg JN, Ring D. Coronoid fracture patterns. J Hand Surg Am 2006;31(1):45–52.
3. Duckworth AD, McQueen MM, Ring D. Fractures of the radial head. Bone Joint J 2013;95-B(2):151–9.
4. Guitton TG, van der Werf HJ, Ring D. Quantitative three-dimensional computed tomography measurement of radial head fractures. J Shoulder Elbow Surg 2010;19(7):973–7.
5. van Leeuwen DH, Guitton TG, Lambers K, et al. Quantitative measurement of radial head fracture location. J Shoulder Elbow Surg 2012;21(8):1013–7.
6. Protzman RR. Dislocation of the elbow joint. J Bone Joint Surg Am 1978;60(4):539–41.
7. Josefsson PO, Gentz CF, Johnell O, et al. Surgical versus non-surgical treatment of ligamentous injuries following dislocation of the elbow joint. A prospective randomized study. J Bone Joint Surg Am 1987;69(4):605–8.
8. Schreiber JJ, Potter HG, Warren RF, et al. Magnetic resonance imaging findings in acute elbow dislocation: insight into mechanism. J Hand Surg Am 2014;39(2):199–205.
9. Papandrea RF, Morrey BF, O'Driscoll SW. Reconstruction for persistent instability of the elbow after coronoid fracture-dislocation. J Shoulder Elbow Surg 2007;16(1):68–77.
10. Lawton JN, Cameron-Donaldson M, Blazar PE, et al. Anatomic considerations regarding the posterior interosseous nerve at the elbow. J Shoulder Elbow Surg 2007;16(4):502–7.
11. Lindenhovius AL, Felsch Q, Ring D, et al. The long-term outcome of open reduction and internal fixation of stable displaced isolated partial articular fractures of the radial head. J Trauma 2009;67(1):143–6.
12. Ring D, Quintero J, Jupiter JB. Open reduction and internal fixation of fractures of the radial head. J Bone Joint Surg Am 2002;84-A(10):1811–5.
13. Wu PH, Shen L, Chee YH. Screw fixation versus arthroplasty versus plate fixation for 3-part radial head fractures. J Orthop Surg (Hong Kong) 2016;24(1):57–61.
14. Shore BJ, Mozzon JB, MacDermid JC, et al. Chronic posttraumatic elbow disorders treated with metallic radial head arthroplasty. J Bone Joint Surg Am 2008;90(2):271–80.
15. Burkhart KJ, Mattyasovszky SG, Runkel M, et al. Mid- to long-term results after bipolar radial head arthroplasty. J Shoulder Elbow Surg 2010;19(7):965–72.
16. Popovic N, Lemaire R, Georis P, et al. Midterm results with a bipolar radial head prosthesis: radiographic evidence of loosening at the bone-cement interface. J Bone Joint Surg Am 2007;89(11):2469–76.
17. Flinkkila T, Kaisto T, Sirnio K, et al. Short- to mid-term results of metallic press-fit radial head arthroplasty in unstable injuries of the elbow. J Bone Joint Surg Br 2012;94(6):805–10.
18. Doornberg JN, Linzel DS, Zurakowski D, et al. Reference points for radial head prosthesis size. J Hand Surg Am 2006;31(1):53–7.
19. Frank SG, Grewal R, Johnson J, et al. Determination of correct implant size in radial head arthroplasty to avoid overlengthening. J Bone Joint Surg Am 2009;91(7):1738–46.
20. Garrigues GE, Wray WH 3rd, Lindenhovius AL, et al. Fixation of the coronoid process in elbow fracture-dislocations. J Bone Joint Surg Am 2011;93(20):1873–81.
21. Ring D, Guss D, Jupiter JB. Reconstruction of the coronoid process using a fragment of discarded radial head. J Hand Surg Am 2012;37(3):570–4.
22. van Riet RP, Morrey BF, O'Driscoll SW. Use of osteochondral bone graft in coronoid fractures. J Shoulder Elbow Surg 2005;14(5):519–23.
23. Moritomo H, Tada K, Yoshida T, et al. Reconstruction of the coronoid for chronic dislocation of the elbow. Use of a graft from the olecranon in two cases. J Bone Joint Surg Br 1998;80(3):490–2.
24. Orbay JL, Mijares MR. The management of elbow instability using an internal joint stabilizer: preliminary results. Clin Orthop Relat Res 2014;472(7):2049–60.
25. Orbay JL, Ring D, Kachooei AR, et al. Multicenter trial of an internal joint stabilizer for the elbow. J Shoulder Elbow Surg 2017;26(1):125–32.
26. McKee MD, Jupiter JB, Bosse G, et al. Outcome of ulnar neurolysis during post-traumatic reconstruction of the elbow. J Bone Joint Surg Br 1998;80(1):100–5.

Arterial Injury in the Upper Extremity
Evaluation, Strategies, and Anticoagulation Management

Cory Lebowitz, DO[a], Jonas L. Matzon, MD[b],*

KEYWORDS

- Upper extremity trauma • Arterial injury • Angiography • Graft • Patency • Anticoagulation

KEY POINTS

- Upper extremity trauma with an associated arterial injury typically occurs via a blunt or penetrating mechanism.
- Given the intricacy of the upper extremity arterial system, the diagnosis of an arterial injury can be challenging and requires a high index of suspicion.
- Appropriate treatment of the arterial injury is dependent on the mechanism and location of the injury.
- Although thrombosis is a common complication of arterial injuries, a standardized anticoagulation regimen has yet to be established.

EPIDEMIOLOGY

Vascular injuries to the extremities account for fewer than 1% of all traumatic injuries, and upper extremity arterial injuries comprise 30% to 40% of all extremity arterial trauma.[1,2] Typically, these injuries are a result of a penetrating or a blunt force mechanism. Although both mechanisms can involve any surrounding tissue, blunt mechanisms are associated with a higher morbidity and mortality due to the more generalized effect of the trauma.[2,3]

With either mechanism, various types of arterial injuries can occur, and these are grouped into 5 types: intimal injury (ie, flaps, disruptions, or subintimal/intramural hematomas), complete wall defect with hemorrhage or pseudoaneurysm, complete transection with hemorrhage or occlusion, arteriovenous fistula, and spasm.[4,5] Penetrating injuries typically cause wall defects. In contrast, blunt trauma usually causes intimal defects via a shearing contusion or crush injury. As a result, focal intimal damage may lead to the formation of an arterial dissection, thrombosis, or a pseudoaneurysm. Injury to a vessel can also be secondary to a stress lesion, such as a dissection or pseudoaneurysm caused by compression of the vessel. Joint dislocation can result in an occlusion or dissection injury. Spasm can occur after either blunt or penetrating trauma to an extremity and is more common in young patients.[5,6]

Upper extremity arterial injuries have the potential to have a substantial impact on the overall outcome for trauma patients. Given that these injuries most commonly affect men from 24 years

Disclosure Statement: None.
[a] Department of Orthopedic Surgery, Rowan University School of Osteopathic Medicine, Stratford, NJ 080084, USA; [b] Department of Orthopaedic Surgery, Thomas Jefferson University, Rothman Institute, 925 Chestnut Street, Philadelphia, PA 19107, USA
* Corresponding author.
E-mail address: jonas.matzon@rothmaninstitute.com

hand.theclinics.com

old to 38 years old, it is understandable how these traumas present difficult medical and socioeconomic problems.[3,5,7] To properly manage these injuries, it is vital to make an appropriate assessment using all tools available.

EVALUATION

The arterial system of the upper extremity begins with the subclavian artery and continues distally as the axillary artery. In turn, this forms the brachial artery, which eventually divides into the radial and ulnar arteries in the forearm. Aside from this typical path, a rich collateral circulation exists (**Fig. 1**).[8] With such an intricate vascular network, the appropriate diagnosis of an arterial injury in an upper extremity trauma patient can be challenging. Specific algorithms can aid the process by providing various subjective and objective tools.

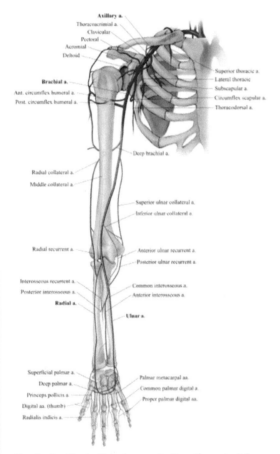

Fig. 1. An illustration demonstrating the arterial system of the upper extremity. a, artery; aa, arteriae. (*From* Daoutis N, Gerostathopoulos N, Bouchlis G, et al. Results after repair of traumatic arterial damage in the forearm. Microsurgery 1992;13(4):176; with permission.)

As with any trauma, the evaluation of a patient with an upper extremity injury begins with the primary survey (ABCDEs according to the Advanced Trauma Life Support protocol: Airway, Breathing, Circulation, Disability and Exposure/Environment).[9] If signs of bleeding are recognized, control by direct compression is advised. In the rare situation where direct compression is unable to provide adequate hemostasis, a tourniquet can be used.[9] Data collected from Operation Enduring Freedom (Afghanistan) and Operation Iraqi Freedom have demonstrated that the appropriate application of a tourniquet is effective in preventing loss of life and is safe, with an overall complication of rate of less than 5%.[9] If a patient's vital signs are unstable, however, immediate resuscitation with blood transfusion is indicated.[9]

Once a patient is hemodynamically stable, the secondary survey is initiated with a detailed history and physical examination focusing on the specific upper extremity injury. Occasionally, the physical examination can be misleading or unimpressive. In fact, 5% to 15% of patients with a vascular injury may present with a normal pulse examination.[5] Therefore, careful attention must be paid to any hard and/or soft signs of vascular trauma (**Table 1**). Hard signs are an absolute indication for vascular exploration, given that these patients have an incidence of vascular injury greater than 90%.[10,11] In contrast, patients with soft signs have an incidence of vascular injury ranging from 3% to 25%.[5]

If there is a high suspicion of vascular injury in the setting of soft signs, numerous noninvasive diagnostic methods have been found helpful (**Fig. 2**). One such diagnostic tool is the arterial pressure index (API), which is the ratio of the

Table 1 **Hard and soft signs of vascular injury in orthopedic trauma**	
"Hard" Signs	**"Soft" Signs**

Pulselessness
Pallor
Paresthesia
Paralysis
Pain
Rapidly expanding
  hematoma
Massive bleeding
Palpable thrill or
  audible bruit
	History of bleeding in
	  transit
	Proximity-related injury
	Neurologic findings
	  from nerve adjacent
	  to a named artery
	Hematoma over a
	  named artery

Data from Doody O, Given M, Lyon S. Extremities—indications and techniques for treatment of extremity vascular injuries. Injury 2008;39(11):1295–303.

definitive vascular repair. These shunts can provide extremity perfusion similar to that of a vascular repair for hours or even days.[20]

Vascular Repair

The technique of achieving definitive arterial perfusion is dependent on the location, mechanism, and severity of arterial damage. During wound exploration, wide exposure is necessary to appropriately visualize the damaged vessel and to adequately obtain proximal and distal control. Occasionally, in cases of difficult exposure, such as the axilla, proximal occlusion can be achieved through the use of a Fogarty balloon catheter. After complete visualization, both ends of the damaged vessel are irrigated with heparinized saline to decrease the risk of thrombosis.[21] The damaged vessel is then assessed for the appropriateness of repair. For short segment injuries (<2 cm), primary repair is optimal if the arterial ends can be mobilized to achieve a tension-free end-to-end anastomosis. After freshening of damaged edges and confirmation of arterial flow from both ends, the repair is accomplished with nonabsorbable, monofilament suture in an interrupted or continuous fashion.[4]

Based on the extent of the vascular injury, primary repair is not always feasible. If resection to healthy intima at both ends results in a long segment gap (>2 cm), primary repair is typically no longer a viable option.[4] In this situation, an autogenous vein graft, an autogenous artery graft, or a synthetic conduit is needed to bridge the gap. The ideal graft should be similar in diameter and vessel wall thickness, readily available, easy to harvest, and have minimal donor site morbidity.[22] In evaluating the use of autogenous vein grafts for arterial repair in injured extremities, Keen and colleagues[23] had an overall limb salvage rate of 97% with primary and secondary patency rates of 99% and 98%, respectively.[23,24] Other studies, however, have reported outcomes with patency ranging from 46% to 85%.[24,25] Depending on the location of the injury, various upper and lower extremity veins have been used as donors.[23] Vein grafts are typically easy to harvest and readily accessible, but they can pose certain challenges in the distal upper extremity. Specifically, veins need to have their valves removed, or the grafts need to be reversed to ensure patency. Valvulotomies are challenging in smaller veins, and reversal often complicates anastomosis, secondary to size mismatch.[22]

Due to these difficulties with vein grafts and the documented success of arterial grafts for cardiac bypass procedures, some surgeons have started using arteries as upper extremity vascular grafts.[22] The benefit of an arterial graft is the increased similarity of the vessel wall anatomy and diameter between native vessel and graft, which can result in improved flow characteristics.[26] Commonly used grafts include the deep inferior epigastric artery, the lateral femoral circumflex artery, and the thoracodorsal artery.[22] Masden and colleagues[24] reviewed multiple studies that reported the use of arterial grafts for distal upper extremity vascular disease (acute and chronic), with patency up to 100%.[24] Although most of these studies were case series and surgical techniques susceptible to selection bias, the use of arterial grafts for upper extremity vascular injury seems a viable option.[24]

Another option for long segment defects is synthetic grafts. Unfortunately, compared with autogenous grafts, synthetic grafts tend to have lower patency rates and higher infection rates.[27] Therefore, synthetic grafts, like polytetrafluoroethylene, are reserved for situations when autogenous graft is not available.[9]

Although open surgical treatment remains the standard of care for peripheral arterial injuries, the continued advancement of radiologic imaging and endovascular surgery has expanded the options in treating traumatic peripheral vascular injuries to include balloon occlusion, embolization, and stent placement.[6,28] Endovascular repair has long been used for less urgent lesions, such as arteriovenous fistula and pseudoaneurysm, and these techniques are now finding their place in emergent care.[2] In some scenarios, endovascular repair can be advantageous over open repair due to its decreased operative time, minimal blood loss, and lower frequency of iatrogenic injuries. Specifically, endovascular repair is becoming more common in treating subclavian and axillary artery injury. These vessels are challenging to explore, and patients with these injuries often present with hemorrhagic shock and anatomic distortion, which often complicates open repair.[28] Worni and colleagues[29] found a lower in-hospital morbidity and mortality for endovascular treatment of peripheral arterial trauma compared with open repair.[29] Although the endovascular management of traumatic arterial injuries seems a viable option, the studies of the technique are limited in numbers and follow-up duration.[28]

Treatment by Location

Shoulder and proximal

Via its blunt mechanism, dislocation is a frequent cause of vascular injury. Scapulothoracic dissociation is the most proximal upper extremity dislocation and also one of the most rare.[2] Patients with scapulothoracic dissociation and an associated arterial injury typically present with a chest wall hematoma, absent pulses, and loss of Doppler signals. Furthermore, these patients often have a concomitant neurologic injury, with an association reported as high as 91%.[2] In contrast, patients with an isolated subclavian artery injury have an associated brachial plexus injury 18% to 33% of the time.[19] These combined injuries result in significant short-term and long-term disability compared with isolated brachial plexus injury.[2] Depending on the severity of arterial injury and the stability of the patient, subclavian arteries can be repaired with any of the previous modalities; however, in the setting of a mangled extremity, primary or secondary amputation remains a consideration.[19]

Unlike scapulothoracic dissociations, uncomplicated shoulder dislocations result in arterial injuries less than 1% of the time.[30] In this scenario, the transection typically occurs from a tethering mechanism that most commonly affects the third part of the axially artery (**Fig. 3**).[31] Unfortunately, physical examination alone is frequently insufficient to rule out arterial disruption, because classic signs of arterial injury may be absent in as many as 40% due to the abundant collateral circulation of the shoulder.[30] When there is concern for possible arterial injury, the shoulder should be reduced rapidly, without prolonging ischemia time.[30] Then, the previously described work-up can be initiated.

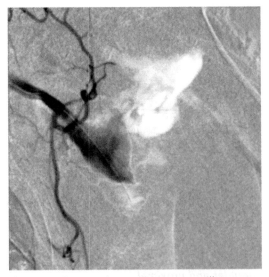

Fig. 3. Angiogram demonstrating an axillary artery transection after a shoulder dislocation. (*From* Ergüneş K, Yazman S, Yetkin U, et al. Axillary artery transection after shoulder dislocation. Ann Vasc Surg 2013;27(7):974.e8; with permission.)

When the axillary artery has been transected, a primary end-to-end repair can often be performed with ligation and division of side branches to enable mobilization of the artery and a tension-free anastomosis.[2] In more complex tears, however, an interposition graft may be required.[2] In contrast, endovascular repair is a reasonable option when the axillary artery is disrupted secondary to pseudoaneurysms, arteriovenous fistulas, branch vessel injuries, intimal flaps, and/or focal lacerations.[31] When there has been minimal soft tissue trauma, even ligation is an option with minimal consequence. When associated with extensive soft tissue trauma, however, there is a high likelihood of collateral disruption leading to a decreased risk of limb survival.[2] Furthermore, axillary artery injuries can have an associated brachial plexus injury secondary to the direct trauma that occurs with a shoulder dislocation. Ergüneş and colleagues[31] reported a 90.4% rate of neurologic injury when the axially artery was transected from a shoulder dislocation.[31] In contrast, the incidence of a brachial plexus injury is 30% to 60% when the axially artery is damaged from a penetrating injury.[32]

Elbow

Closed elbow injuries, such as pediatric supracondylar humerus fractures and uncomplicated elbow dislocation, have the potential to disrupt the brachial artery.[30] In fact, 4% of patients with pediatric supracondylar humerus fractures present with a pale, pulseless hand.[33] In this scenario, skeletal stabilization is initially performed. After closed reduction percutaneous pinning (CRPP) of the fracture, 37% of patients have return of capillary refill and only 5% require vascular exploration.[33] Patients displaying signs of perfusion (ie, pink hand) with pulses after CRPP can be safely observed.[21] In contrast, patients with persistence of a poorly perfused, pulseless extremity after CRPP require immediate vascular exploration (**Fig. 4**).[34] There remains controversy, however, whether to observe or explore patients with a pulseless but perfused extremity after CRPP.[34]

If the brachial artery is injured, it can be treated with any of the previously discussed techniques. End-to-end anastomosis is preferable if it can be performed without tension or damage to major collateral vessels, but higher-energy mechanisms are more likely to require repair with a graft.[2,12] Moreover, traumatic brachial artery injuries have associated complications and injuries. Kim and colleagues[35] reported an approximately 20% incidence of compartment syndrome requiring fasciotomy in patients with a brachial artery

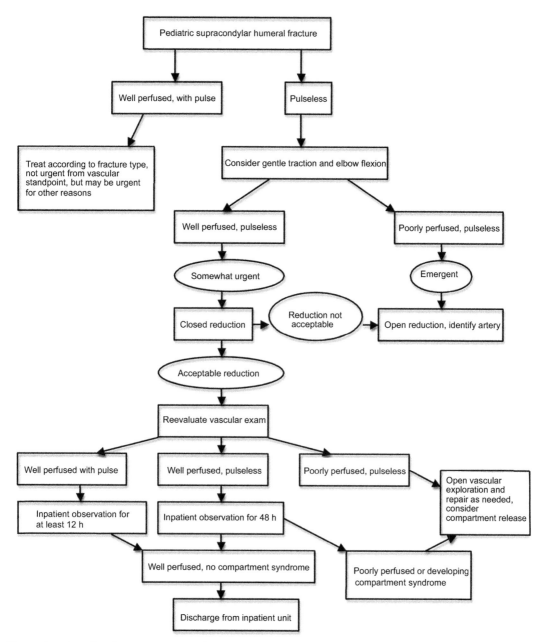

Fig. 4. Flowchart for the management of an extremity with or without vascular compromise in the setting of a pediatric supracondylar humerus fracture. (*From* Badkoobehi H, Choi PD, Bae DS, et al. Management of the pulseless pediatric supracondylar humeral fracture. J Bone Joint Surg Am 2015;97(11):940; with permission.)

injury.[35] Furthermore, associated nerve injuries are common with an approximate incidence of 25%, and the median nerve is the most frequently affected compared with the radial and ulnar nerves.[12] These associated injuries often limit the function of the affected upper extremity even after successful arterial repair and lead to a 36% chance of long-term disability.[12]

Forearm/wrist

Penetrating injuries to the radial and/or ulnar artery in the forearm and wrist are typically the result of lacerations by knife, glass, or machinery. Initially, hemorrhage is controlled by means of direct compression. Subsequently, a thorough physical examination should focus on the nearby muscles, tendons, and nerves, because these are commonly injured.[36,37] Although a patient typically presents with ischemia in the setting of an injury to both the radial and ulnar arteries, ischemia rarely results from a single-artery injury. This is true even in the 20% of the population who have an incomplete palmar arch, due to the intact collaterals between the radial and ulnar arteries.[37] As discussed previously, patients with hard signs are brought to the operating room emergently. Forearm arterial repairs in a well-perfused hand, however, have showed no difference in functional outcome when taken to the operating room emergently (within 6 hours) or in a delayed manner.[38]

Surgical treatment of arterial injuries in the forearm can be accomplished with repair or ligation. When there is no distal perfusion, repair is the treatment of choice. Gelberman and colleagues[39] proposed that immediate repair of both vessels be attempted when both the radial and ulnar arteries are damaged and there is distal ischemia.[39] In the situation where both arteries are injured yet distal perfusion seems adequate, operative repair of both vessels is still recommended to lessen the chance that ischemic symptoms will occur.[17,39] In the setting of single-artery damage (either radial or ulnar) with intact perfusion of the hand, however, ligation versus repair is a topic of debate.[40] Due to the substantial collateral network throughout the forearm and hand, ligation is considered an acceptable option.[3] First, it has economic benefits because fewer resources are required in comparison to repair.[40] Furthermore, Johnson[37] found no instances of claudication with ligation of a single vessel; however, hand weakness (50%) and cold insensitivity (12%) were noted in those with a concomitant nerve injury.[37] In contrast, Basseto and colleagues[40] reported greater loss of bone mass, muscular mass, and strength in patients who had undergone arterial ligation without an associated nerve damage; hence, they advocated for surgical repair even in single-vessel damage in the setting of perfusion.[40]

Although both surgical ligation and primary repair can be reasonable choices after forearm arterial injuries, neither option is without complication. Ligating a vessel or failure of repair can result in acute-on-chronic ischemia. This scenario has occurred after an acute traumatic event in patients with a remote history of radial forearm flaps, where the radial artery harvest is the source of chronic disease. Due to adequate collateral blood flow, the harvest may never show signs of ischemia until an acute traumatic event.[41] In primary repairs, claudication, ischemia, and/or cold intolerance are usually related with the patency of repair.[42] Patency rates for an individual radial or ulnar artery repair with use of microsurgical technique is

reported between 46%[37] and 77%.[43] Patency can also be complicated by thrombosis, which occurs from stasis and reduced flow, likely secondary to the high retrograde pressure in the distal arterial stump from incompleteness of the arches.[39] For this reason, Gelberman and colleagues[39] advocate for single-vessel repair because some patients may have incomplete arches.[39] Early repairs within 36 hours, sharp lacerations (i,e not crush or avulsion injuries), and radial repairs (when compared with ulnar) have demonstrated higher patency rates.[39] Due to the potential of thrombosis, it is recommended that repairs be assessed both clinically and diagnostically to correlate clinical symptomatology and patency rates. This can be performed via Doppler ultrasound and/or angiography.[43]

Hand

Acute arterial injuries to the hand and finger are commonly the result of a penetrating mechanism and are frequently work related.[44] Arterial injuries distal to the forearm are frequently accompanied by an associated nerve, tendon, bone, and soft tissue damage. Single digital artery injuries rarely result in loss of distal perfusion, and, therefore, they do not necessitate treatment in isolation. When both digital arteries of a finger are injured, however, the treatment algorithm is complex due to the severity of associated injuries. Surgical options include amputation, revascularization, replantation, flap coverage, skin graft coverage, and others.[45] Each technique has specific indications, but a review of the various options is beyond the scope of this article.

ANTICOAGULATION MANAGEMENT

Besides adequate acute intervention, successful treatment of upper extremity arterial injuries requires appropriate postinjury management. Unlike the standardized anticoagulation/antiaggregant therapy for thrombus prophylaxis in chronic vascular disease, the literature on the use of anticoagulation for the management of acute upper extremity arterial injury is scarce. Although surgeons have documented anticoagulation protocols based on their training and anecdotal experience, few data exist to support one method over another **(Table 3)**.[9,12,21,46–56]

Although a standard protocol for anticoagulation does not exist when managing upper extremity arterial injuries, Conrad and Adams[57] made recommendations for the use of antithrombotics in managing free flaps and replants. They recommended the use of aspirin for 2 weeks postoperatively, heparin as an intraoperative saline irrigant,

Table 3
Summary of recent anticoagulation use for upper extremity arterial injuries and their associated treatment

Study	Pathology	Repair	Anticoagulation
Mehlhoff and Wood,[47] 1991	Ulnar artery thrombosis	Venous graft	Aspirin 325 mg tid dipyridamole 3 wk
Barral et al,[48] 1992	Posttraumatic arterial lesion, embolism, aneurysm	Palmar bypass: radiopalmar, ulnarpalmar, distal radial bypass, palmopalmar	Ticlopidine 3 mo subcutaneous heparin 15 d
Nehler et al,[49] 1992	Distal to the wrist	Arterial bypass	Nothing
Zimmerman et al,[50] 1994	Ulnar artery occlusion	Ligation, arterial reconstruction	LMW dextran 72 h, then aspirin 325 mg for 6 mo
Ruch et al,[51] 2000	Radial artery occlusion near the carpus	Vein graft	LMW dextran for 72 h, then aspirin 325 mg for 6 wk
Smith et al,[52] 2004	Hypothenar hammer syndrome	Autologous inferior epigastric artery	Continuous infusion of diltiazem at 15 mg/h and dextran for 24 h after surgery followed by diltiazem
Shalabi et al,[53] 2006	UE injury: subclavian, axillary, brachial, radial, ulnar artery	EEA, venous interposition graft, ligation	PO IV heparin 5–7 d and discharged on oral aspirin 100 mg tablet/d for 12 wk
Ergünes et al,[12] 2006	Brachial artery injury	Primary repair, SVIG	Systemic and intraoperative heparin (with PO systemic heparin patients with graft and soft tissue injury
Carrafiello et al,[54] 2011	UE injury: subclavian, axillary, brachial artery	Bare stent, percutaenous transluminal angioplasty, stent graft	PO 0.7 IU of LMW heparin bid for 30 d with lifelong 120 mg/d ticlopidine or acetylsalicylic acid
Temming et al,[55] 2011	Ulnar artery thrombosis hypothenar hammer syndrome	Descending branch of the lateral circumflex femoral artery graft	Aspirin 100 mg for 2 wk
Krishnan et al,[56] 2014	Upper and lower extremity arterial injury	SVIG, polytetrafluoroethylene	Dextran-40 for first 24 h followed by subcutaneous LMW heparin for a week. Discharged on 6-wk aspirin (150 mg daily)
Ivatury et al,[9] 2014	Penetrating extremity arterial Injury	Primary, EEA, autogenous graft, prosthetic Graft	Intraoperative systemic heparin and local heparin

Abbreviations: bid, 2 times a day; EEA, end-to-end anastamosis; d, day; h, hour; IO, intraoperative; IV, intravenous; LMW, low molecular weight; PO, postoperative; SVIG, saphenous vein interposition graft; tid, 3 times a day; UE, upper extremity; wk, week.

and a heparin bolus (50–100 U/kg) before releasing the clamps. For replants, they also recommended dextran-40 at 0.4 mL/kg/h, which was weaned off by postoperative day 5.[58] Given the similarity in arterial repair, their protocol could potentially be extrapolated to upper extremity arterial injuries.

Overall, anticoagulation use is prevalent in the management of upper extremity arterial injuries to prevent thrombosis and protect the patency of repair. Although these agents have theoretic use, well-supported clinical evidence is needed to formulate standardized guidelines.

TREATMENT OUTCOME

Upper extremity arterial injuries may present alone or with a magnitude of associated injuries. Although various factors contribute to the outcome, the presence of an associated neurologic injury is associated with long-term morbidity. Patients with an associated nerve injury have a 27% to 44% rate of functional disability.[9,12] To minimize this risk, it is recommended that nerve injuries be repaired as early as possible.[3] Apart from recognizing an associated neurologic injury, early detection of graft failure, compartment syndrome, and infection also dramatically improve patient outcome.[7]

Upper extremity arterial injuries can present in myriad ways. Managing these injuries likely requires the assistance of multiple medical teams, with a goal to first preserve life and then limb. Overall, with the adjunct of thorough diagnostic tools, increased availability of resources, and an aggressive philosophy of surgical intervention, limb salvage rates are high (92% to 100%) and mortality rates are low (0% to 24%).[4]

REFERENCES

1. Diamond S, Gaspard D, Katz S. Vascular injuries to the extremities in a suburban trauma center. Am Surg 2003;69:848–51.
2. Baker AC, Clouse WD. Upper extremity and junctional zone injuries. Rich's Vascular Trauma. 2016. p. 149–167.
3. Franz RW, Goodwin RB, Hartman JF, et al. Management of upper extremity arterial injuries at an urban level I trauma center. Ann Vasc Surg 2009;23(1):8–16.
4. Franz RW, Skytta CK, Shah KJ, et al. A five-year review of management of upper-extremity arterial injuries at an urban level I trauma center. Ann Vasc Surg 2012;26(5):655–64.
5. Mavrogenis AF, Panagopoulos GN, Kokkalis ZT, et al. Vascular Injury in Orthopedic Trauma. Orthopedics 2016;39(4):249–59.
6. Doody O, Given M, Lyon S. Extremities—indications and techniques for treatment of extremity vascular injuries. Injury 2008;39(11):1295–303.
7. Dragas M, Davidovic L, Kostic D, et al. Upper extremity arterial injuries: factors influencing treatment outcome. Injury 2009;40(8):815–9.
8. Doyle JR, Botte MJ. Surgical anatomy of the hand and upper extremity. Philadelphia: Lippincott Williams & Wilkins; 2003.
9. Ivatury RR, Anand R, Ordonez C. Penetrating extremity trauma. World J Surg 2014;39(6):1389–96.
10. Ascher E, Haimovici H. Haimovici's vascular surgery. Malden (MA): Blackwell Pub; 2004.
11. Feliciano DV. Management of peripheral arterial injury. Curr Opin Crit Care 2010;16(6):602–8.
12. Ergünes K, Yilik L, Ozsoyler I, et al. Traumatic brachial artery injuries. Tex Heart Inst J 2006;33: 31–4.
13. Bravman JT, Ipaktchi K, Biffl WL, et al. Vascular injuries after minor blunt upper extremity trauma: pitfalls in the recognition and diagnosis of potential "near miss" injuries. Scand J Trauma Resusc Emerg Med 2008;16(1):1–6.
14. Soto JA, Múnera F, Morales C, et al. Focal arterial injuries of the proximal extremities: helical CT arteriography as the initial method of diagnosis. Radiology 2001;218(1):188–94.
15. Jens S, Kerstens M, Legemate D, et al. Diagnostic performance of computed tomography angiography in peripheral arterial injury due to trauma: a systematic review and meta-analysis. J Vasc Surg 2013; 58(3):846–7.
16. Fritz J, Efron DT, Fishman EK. Multidetector CT and three-dimensional CT angiography of upper extremity arterial injury. Emerg Radiol 2014;22(3):269–82.
17. Daoutis N, Gerostathopoulos N, Bouchlis G, et al. Results after repair of traumatic arterial damage in the forearm. Microsurgery 1992;13(4):175–7.
18. Prichayudh S, Verananvattna A, Sriussadaporn S, et al. Management of upper extremity vascular injury: outcome related to the mangled extremity severity score. World J Surg 2009;33(4):857–63.
19. Slauterbeck JR, Britton C, Moneim MS, et al. Mangled extremity severity score: an accurate guide to treatment of the severely injured upper extremity. J Orthop Trauma 1994;8(4):282–5.
20. Gifford SM, Aidinian G, Clouse WD, et al. Effect of temporary shunting on extremity vascular injury: an outcome analysis from the Global War on Terror vascular injury initiative. J Vasc Surg 2009;50(3): 549–56.
21. Pederson WC. Acute ischemia of the upper extremity. Orthop Clin North Am 2016;47(3):589–97.
22. Trocchia AM, Hammert WC. Arterial grafts for vascular reconstruction in the upper extremity. J Hand Surg 2011;36(9):1534–6.
23. Keen RR, Meyer JP, Durham JR, et al. Autogenous vein graft repair of injured extremity arteries: early and late results with 134 consecutive patients. J Vasc Surg 1991;13(5):664–8.
24. Masden D, Seruya M, Higgins JP. A systematic review of distal upper extremity bypass surgery: a comparison o arterial and venous conduits. J Hand Surg 2012;37(8):36.
25. Lannau B, Bliley J, James IB, et al. Long-term patency of primary arterial repair and the modified cold intolerance symptom severity questionnaire. Plast Reconstr Surg Glob Open 2015;3(11):e551.
26. Cooper GJ, Underwood MJ, Deverall PB. Arterial and venous conduits for coronary artery bypass. A current review. Eur J Cardiothorac Surg 1996; 10(2):129–40.
27. Yavuz S, Tiryakioglu O, Celkan A, et al. Emergency surgical procedures in the peripheral vascular injuries. Turk J Vasc Surg 2000;1:15–20.

28. Scott AR, Gilani R, Tapia NM, et al. Endovascular management of traumatic peripheral arterial injuries. J Surg Res 2015;199(2):557–63.

29. Worni M, Scarborough JE, Gandhi M, et al. Use of endovascular therapy for peripheral arterial lesions: an analysis of the national trauma data bank from 2007 to 2009. Ann Vasc Surg 2013;27(3):299–305.

30. Sparks SR, Delarosa J, Bergan JJ, et al. Arterial injury in uncomplicated upper extremity dislocations. Ann Vasc Surg 2000;14(2):110–3.

31. Ergüneş K, Yazman S, Yetkin U, et al. Axillary artery transection after shoulder dislocation. Ann Vasc Surg 2013;27(7):974.e7-10.

32. Gill H, Jenkins W, Edu S, et al. Civilian penetrating axillary artery injuries. World J Surg 2011;35(5):962–6.

33. Weller A, Garg S, Larson AN, et al. Management of the pediatric pulseless supracondylar humeral fracture: is vascular exploration necessary? J Bone Joint Surg Am 2013;95(21):1906–12.

34. Badkoobehi H, Choi PD, Bae DS, et al. Management of the pulseless pediatric supracondylar humeral fracture. J Bone Joint Surg Am 2015;97(11):937–43.

35. Kim JYS, Buck DW, Forte AJV, et al. Risk factors for compartment syndrome in traumatic brachial artery injuries: an Institutional experience in 139 patients. J Trauma 2009;67(6):1339–44.

36. Thai J, Pacheco J, Margolis D, et al. Evidence-based comprehensive approach to forearm arterial laceration. West J Emerg Med 2015;16(7):1127–34.

37. Johnson M. Radial or ulnar artery laceration. Arch Surg 1993;128(9):971.

38. Park MJ, Gans I, Lin I, et al. Timing of forearm arterial repair in the well-perfused limb. Orthopedics 2014;37(6):582–6.

39. Gelberman RH, Nunley JA, Koman LA, et al. The results of radial and ulnar arterial repair in the forearm. Experience in three medical centers. J Bone Joint Surg 1982;64(3):383–7.

40. Bassetto F, Zucchetto M, Vindigni V, et al. Traumatic musculoskeletal changes in forearm and hand after emergency vascular anastomosis or ligation. J Reconstr Microsurg 2010;26(07):441–7.

41. Higgins JP. A reassessment of the role of the radial forearm flap in upper extremity reconstruction. J Hand Surg 2011;36(7):1237–40.

42. Nunley JA, Goldner RD, Koman LA, et al. Arterial stump pressure: a determinant of arterial patency? J Hand Surg 1987;12(2):245–9.

43. Bacakoğlu ACBC, Özkan MH, Coşkunol E, et al. Multifactorial effects on the patency rates of forearm arterial repairs. Microsurgery 2001;21(2):37–42.

44. Sorock GS, Lombardi DA, Hauser RB, et al. Acute traumatic occupational hand injuries: type, location, and severity. J Occup Environ Med 2002;44(4):345–51.

45. Christoforou D, Alaia M, Craig-Scott S. Microsurgical management of acute traumatic injuries of the hand and fingers. Bull Hosp Jt Dis 2013;71(1):6–16.

46. Xipoleas G, Levine E, Silver L, et al. A survey of microvascular protocols for lower extremity free tissue transfer II. Ann Plast Surg 2008;61(3): 280–4.

47. Mehlhoff TL, Wood MB. Ulnar artery thrombosis and the role of interposition vein grafting: Patency with microsurgical technique. J Hand Surg 1991;16(2): 274–8.

48. Barral X, Favre JP, Gournier JP, et al. Late results of palmar arch bypass in the treatment of digital trophic disorders. Ann Vasc Surg 1992;6(5):418–24.

49. Nehler MR, Dalman RL, Harris E, et al. Upper extremity arterial bypass distal to the wrist. J Vasc Surg 1992;16(4):633–42.

50. Zimmerman NB, Zimmerman SI, Mcclinton MA, et al. Long-term recovery following surgical treatment for ulnar artery occlusion. J Hand Surg 1994;19(1):17–21.

51. Ruch DS, Aldridge M, Holden M, et al. Arterial reconstruction for radial artery occlusion. J Hand Surg 2000;25(2):282–90.

52. Smith HE, Dirks M, Patterson RB. Hypothenar hammer syndrome: distal ulnar artery reconstruction with autologous inferior epigastric artery. J Vasc Surg 2004;40(6):1238–42.

53. Shalabi R, Amri YA, Khoujah E. Vascular injuries of the upper extremity. J Vasc Bras 2006;5(4):271–6.

54. Carrafiello G, Laganà D, Mangini M, et al. Percutaneous treatment of traumatic upper-extremity arterial injuries: a single-center experience. J Vasc Interv Radiol 2011;22(1):34–9.

55. Temming JF, Uchelen JHV, Tellier MA. Hypothenar hammer syndrome. Tech Hand Up Extrem Surg 2011;15(1):24–7.

56. Krishnan J, Paiman M, Nawfar A, et al. The outcomes of salvage surgery for vascular injury in the extremities: a special consideration for delayed revascularization. Malays Orthop J 2014;8(1):14–20.

57. Conrad MH, Adams WP. Pharmacologic optimization of microsurgery in the new millennium. Plast Reconstr Surg 2001;108(7):2088–97.

58. Askari M, Fisher C, Weniger FG, et al. Anticoagulation therapy in microsurgery: a review. J Hand Surg 2006;31(5):836–46.

Ulnar Nerve Management with Distal Humerus Fracture Fixation: A Meta-Analysis

CrossMark

Jonathan W. Shearin, MD[a], Talia R. Chapman, MD[b],*,
Andrew Miller, MD[b], Asif M. Ilyas, MD[c]

KEYWORDS

• Humerus • Internal fixation • Ulnar nerve • Meta-analysis • Transposition • Decompression

KEY POINTS

• Ulnar neuropathy is common after distal humerus fracture repair surgery, with an overall incidence of 19% postoperatively.
• The ulnar nerve is typically managed intraoperatively with in situ neurolysis or transposition during fracture fixation.
• Postoperative ulnar neuropathy was increased in patients who underwent transposition versus in situ management of the ulnar nerve.
• It is unclear if the higher prevalence of neuropathy in cases with a transposition is due to greater fracture severity, iatrogenic injury during dissection or transposition, or subsequent postsurgical scarring with fracture healing. However, the authors can conclude transposition does not have a protective effect against the development of late ulnar neuropathy after distal humerus fracture repair surgery.

INTRODUCTION

Fractures of the elbow account for approximately 7% of adult fractures,[1] and distal humerus fractures comprise 30% of all elbow fractures.[2] When open reduction and internal fixation (ORIF) is indicated, several operative complications such as nonunion, loss of functional motion, and ulnar neuropathy have been reported.[3,4] Sodergard and colleagues[5] discussed complications following ORIF of distal humerus fractures, including fixation failure, nerve injury, and infection. Furthermore, Gofton and colleagues[6] reported complication rates up to 48%, which included heterotopic ossification (17%), infection (9%), and olecranon nonunion (9%).

Ulnar neuropathy in particular poses a unique challenge, as it can be a product of the initial injury, surgical management, or postoperative rehabilitation. The rate of ulnar neuropathy following ORIF of distal humerus fractures has been reported between 0% and 51% in previously described studies.[7,8] It is currently not well understood what the best method is for managing the ulnar nerve during ORIF between leaving the nerve in situ or transposing it.

Huang and colleagues[8] conducted a retrospective evaluation of distal humerus fractures treated operatively at a level 1 trauma center between 1997 and 2005 in patients older than 65 years. At the final follow-up (range 20–99 months), the

Disclosure Statement: The authors have no relevant disclosures.
[a] Hand & Upper Extremity Surgery, Department of Orthopedic Surgery, Arnot Health, Elmira, NY, USA;
[b] Department of Orthopedic Surgery, Thomas Jefferson University Hospital, 1025 Walnut Street, Suite 516, Philadelphia, PA 19107, USA; [c] Department of Orthopedic Surgery, Rothman Institute at Thomas Jefferson University, 925 Chestnut, Philadelphia, PA 19107, USA
* Corresponding author.
E-mail address: Talia.chapman10@gmail.com

Hand Clin 34 (2018) 97–103
https://doi.org/10.1016/j.hcl.2017.09.010
0749-0712/18/© 2017 Elsevier Inc. All rights reserved.

hand.theclinics.com

mean Mayo Elbow Performance score was 83 (range 55–100) with 6 excellent (95–100), 3 good (75–90), 3 fair (60–74), and 2 poor (less than 60) results. They reported a postoperative rate of ulnar neuropathy of 0%.

Similarly, Doornberg and colleagues[9] conducted a retrospective study looking at 30 adult patients who underwent operative treatment of complete articular fractures of the distal humerus. The average age of this cohort was 35 years. The average length of the follow-up was 19 years (range 12–35 years). They used multiple surveys to assess functional outcomes. Ultimately, they found that at the follow-up, the average flexion arc was greater than 100°, the average Disabilities of Arm, Shoulder, and Hands (DASH) score was comparable with the average score in the general US population and that arthrosis was present in most (80%) of the patients; these outcomes were not independent predictors of patient-rated disability (DASH score) or surgeon-rated elbow function. They also described only a 3% rate of postoperative ulnar neuropathy.

On the other hand, Vazquez and colleagues[10] retrospectively evaluated 69 distal humerus bicolumnar fractures treated with ORIF. In 47 patients, the nerve was left anterior in the subcutaneous tissues; in the remainder of the patients, it was placed back in the cubital tunnel. They reported 14 patients with documented ulnar nerve dysfunction at either the immediate postoperative period or at the final evaluation. In the immediate postoperative period, 7 patients had neuropathy and 4 had been transposed. In 3 of these patients, symptoms resolved at the 1-year point; but 7 additional patients developed neuropathy and, among those, 5 had been transposed. Ultimately, there was no significant difference between the two strategies of handling the ulnar nerve and the development of ulnar neuropathy.

Chen and colleagues[11] performed a retrospective review of 137 consecutive patients who underwent ORIF of an Orthopedic Trauma Association 13A or 13C distal humerus fracture by one of 3 orthopedic trauma surgeons at 2 institutions between 1996 and 2005. Two cohorts were identified: 89 patients (mean age 48.6 years) who had not undergone an ulnar nerve transposition and 48 patients (mean age 43.2 years) who had undergone a transposition during ORIF. The decision for transposition was based on surgeon preference and implant position. They found that symptoms of ulnar neuritis occurred 4 times more frequently in patients who had undergone transposition. The incidence of postoperative ulnar neuritis in patients who had undergone transposition was 16 of 48 (33%) and only 8 of 89

(9%) in patients who underwent in situ decompression. Based on this study, the investigators do not recommend routine transposition of the ulnar nerve at the time of ORIF of distal humerus fractures.

Ruan and colleagues[12] evaluated 117 consecutive patients who sustained an Arbeitsgemeinschaft für Osteosynthesefragen (AO) type C fracture of the distal humerus and were treated with ORIF. They found that 29 of the patients (24.8%) presented with ulnar nerve symptoms before operative treatment. They then divided that cohort into 2 groups: one group received ORIF in conjunction with anterior subfascial transposition of the ulnar nerve and the other group received ORIF in conjunction with in situ decompression. All patients were followed up for an average of 29.5 months postoperatively, and all fractures healed appropriately. They found that in the transposition group, 12 of 15 patients recovered completely and 3 patients recovered partially. In the in situ decompression group, they found that 8 of 14 nerves recovered completely and 6 patients recovered partially. They concluded that transposition of the nerve may have benefits with respect to postoperative recovery of nerve function.

In the Canadian Orthopedic Trauma Society's randomized trial of ORIF versus total elbow arthroplasty for bicolumnar fractures of the distal humerus, 20 patients were randomized to receive ORIF and 20 were randomized to receive total elbow arthroplasty (TEA). Five of the patients randomized to the ORIF group were converted intraoperatively to TEA. They routinely transposed the ulnar nerve in both cohorts and reported that the rate of postoperative ulnar nerve symptoms was 20% (5 patients in the ORIF group and 3 in the TEA group).[3]

Worden and Ilyas[13] conducted a retrospective chart review of all patients aged 18 years and older who underwent ORIF for a distal humerus fracture between 2004 and 2008 at a level I urban academic medical center. Patients were excluded if they had a preinjury history of ulnar nerve dysfunction. The ulnar nerve was either managed with an in situ release or anterior transposition. McGowan[14] staging was used to assess the severity of ulnar nerve dysfunction. Grade I was defined as minimal lesions with no motor weakness of the ulnar intrinsics and paresthesia in the ulnar nerve distribution. Grade II was defined as intermediate lesions with weak interossei and decreased sensation. Grade III was defined as a severe lesion with interossei paralysis and marked hypoesthesia. They included 24 cases and found that 50% of the cases had undergone in situ release and 50% were anteriorly transposed. Ultimately, they reported a 38% incidence of postoperative ulnar neuropathy in surgically treated distal humerus fractures with 55% graded as McGowan stage 1 and 44% McGowan stage 2. Among the patients with persistent ulnar neuropathy at the final follow-up, 44% (4) had undergone an in situ release and 56% (5) had undergone an anterior transposition. This difference was not statistically significant.

Wang and colleagues[15] evaluated 20 patients with distal intracondylar humerus fractures treated with dual-plate internal fixation and anterior subcutaneous transposition of the ulnar nerve between 1986 and 1990. Olecranon osteotomy was used in all cases. The average age of the cohort was 47 years, and the average follow-up was 26 months. They described 75% of patients attained excellent or good results. They reported no cases of postoperative nerve compression symptoms in the follow-up period.

Lastly, Holdsworth and Mossad[7] reviewed 57 adult patients at an average of 37 months after early internal fixation for displaced fractures of the distal humerus from 1980 to 1986. The surgical approach was varied based on the type of fracture. They reported an incidence of 50% of postoperative ulnar neuropathy, but they noted only 2 patients with symptoms at the latest follow-up.

Despite this relatively high and somewhat varied prevalence, there is no clear consensus regarding the best method for managing the ulnar nerve during ORIF. Given the paucity and contradictory nature of the data, the authors set out to perform a meta-analysis to evaluate whether a best method exists for handling the ulnar nerve, specifically whether in situ management versus transposition results in a lower incidence of postoperative ulnar neuropathy. As a secondary goal, the authors attempted to evaluate whether the hardware location also influenced postoperative ulnar neuropathy.

METHODS

The guidelines set forth by the Preferred Reporting Items for Systematic Reviews and Meta-analyses guided the authors' investigation. The articles were judged based on the following aspects: (1) equality of baseline characteristics, (2) adequate description of inclusion/exclusion criteria and interventions, (3) validity of outcome tools, (4) duration of follow-up, and (5) primary outcome measure. Specifically, studies that reported on the management of the ulnar nerve in distal humerus fracture fixation were included. The main operative treatments had to be distal humerus fracture ORIF. The management of the ulnar nerve had to be documented and then categorized as either in situ or transposition. The following database was

searched: PubMed MEDLINE (1950 through March 2016). The search strategy involved the terms *distal humerus*, *open reduction internal fixation*, and *ulnar nerve*. A total of 46 studies were identified by the initial search and assessed. Studies that did not report on how the ulnar nerve was handled or did not report on patients' symptoms as related to the ulnar nerve postoperatively were excluded, yielding 5 studies for inclusion. Also, studies discussing the management of distal humerus fractures with arthroplasty were also excluded. Extracted data from the eligible studies included patient characteristics, sample size, fracture type, length of follow-up, surgical fixation, intraoperative management of the ulnar nerve, and outcomes related to ulnar nerve function. The weighted effect size was calculated (Cohen D) and used as it pertained to in situ versus transposition as well as the presence or absence of a medial plate. Cohen D is an effect size that is used to indicate the standardized difference between 2 means. It expresses this difference of specified means in standard deviation units.

RESULTS

All 5 included studies on distal humerus fractures treated with ORIF with either in situ management or anterior transposition reported on postoperative symptoms of ulnar neuropathy. Study characteristics can be seen in **Table 1**. All 5 studies were retrospective studies, totaling 366 distal humerus fracture cases that underwent ORIF and either ulnar nerve in situ management or anterior transposition. In total, 187 patients were treated with in situ management, whereas 179 underwent transposition. The incidence of ulnar neuritis based on handling of the ulnar nerve can be seen in **Table 1**. The overall incidence of ulnar neuropathy in all cases included in the meta-analysis was 19.3% (range 16%–37% in 362 cases). The meta-analysis found that the incidence of neuropathy in the transposition group was higher (23.5%) as compared with the in situ group (15.3%).

Ruan and colleagues[12] demonstrated that of their 29 patients with type C distal humerus fractures and preoperative ulnar nerve symptoms who underwent ORIF, 3 of the 15 ulnar nerves that were transposed did not recover. Of the 14 that underwent in situ management, 6 continued to have postoperative ulnar neuropathy. Vazquez and colleagues[10] demonstrated in their cohort of type A and type C distal humerus fractures that 7 of 47 patients undergoing transposition developed postoperative ulnar neuritis, whereas 4 of 18 developed neuropathy after in situ management. Worden and Ilyas[13] showed that 5 of 12 patients

Table 1
Characteristics of the studies included in the meta-analysis

Study, Year	In Situ	Transposed	Postoperative Ulnar Neuritis	AO Fracture Classification
Ruan et al, 2009	14	15	3 of 15 Patients with transposition 6 of 14 Patients with in situ management	117 Patients type C
Vazquez et al,[10] 2010	22	47	7 of 47 Patients with transposition 4 of 18 Patients with in situ management	69 Patients type A or C
Worden and Ilyas,[13] 2012	12	12	5 of 12 Patients with transposition 4 of 12 Patients with in situ management	7 Patients AO type A, 2 type B, 15 type C
Chen et al,[11] 2010	89	48	16 of 48 Patients with transposition 8 of 89 Patients with in situ management	4 Patients type A2, 4 type A3, 18 type C1, 61 type C2, 50 type C3
Wiggers et al,[16] 2012	50	57	11 of 57 Patients with transposition 6 of 50 Patients with in situ management	12 Patients type A, 46 type B, 49 type C

who underwent transposition developed postoperative ulnar neuritis and, similarly, 4 of 12 patients who were managed in situ developed postoperative neuropathy. Worden and Ilyas[13] included all types of distal humerus fractures (AO type A, B, C). In a slightly larger cohort, Chen and colleagues[11] described an incidence of postoperative ulnar neuritis in 16 of 48 patients who underwent transposition and 8 of 89 patients who underwent in situ management. All types of distal humerus fractures were included. Lastly, Wiggers and colleagues[16] demonstrated in their cohort of all types of distal humerus fractures that 11 of 57 patients who underwent transposition developed neuritis, whereas 6 of 50 who underwent in situ decompression developed postoperative ulnar neuropathy.

Of the available data from Wiggers and colleagues[16] and Worden and Ilyas,[13] the authors ascertained that, in total, 83 patients underwent medial plating and 23 of these developed postoperative ulnar neuritis: 14 of 62 in the Wiggers and colleagues[16] cohort developed ulnar neuropathy and 9 of 21 in the Worden and Ilyas[13] cohort.

The weighted effect size was calculated (Cohen D) in **Table 2** and used to determine the chance that a person picked at random from the treatment group (transposition group) versus the control group (in situ release) will have a higher incidence of ulnar neuropathy. Similarly, the weighted effect

size was calculated (Cohen D) in **Table 2** and used to determine if the presence of a medial plate affected the incidence of postoperative ulnar neuropathy. A calculated weighted effect size (Cohen D value) of 0.427 was interpreted for handling of the ulnar nerve as follows: 66% of the transposition group will be greater than the mean as compared with the control group and, therefore, will have a higher incidence of ulnar neuropathy and 84% of the 2 groups will overlap. There is a 61% chance that a person picked at random from the transposition group will have a higher incidence of ulnar neuropathy as compared with the control group. Furthermore, in order to have an unfavorable outcome in the treatment group, at least 8 people need to be transposed; if 100 people undergo treatment with transposition or in situ management, 13 more patients will experience ulnar neuropathy in the transposition group than in the in situ group.

A weighted effect size (Cohen D value) of 0.6 was calculated and interpreted for the placement of a medial plate and its effect on postoperative ulnar neuropathy. Seventy-three percent of the group receiving a medial plate will be greater than the mean of the control group (no medial plate). There is a 66% chance that a person picked at random from the treatment group (medial plate group) will have an incidence of ulnar neuropathy compared with a person picked at random from

Table 2
Calculated weighted effect size for transposition versus in situ management of the ulnar nerve and for medial plating of distal humerus fractures

Transposition vs Nontransposition	Effect Size Calculations			
	Individual Effect Size (d)	Correlation	Sample Size	Individual Effect Size (d)
Ruan et al,[12] 2009	0.89	0.41	29	0.89
Chen et al,[11] 2010	0.62	0.3	137	0.62
Vazquez et al,[10] 2010	0.26	0.13	69	0.26
Worden and Ilyas,[13] 2012	0.49	0.24	24	0.49
Wiggers et al,[16] 2012	0.15	0.07	107	0.15
	Weighted effect size (Cohen D) 0.427			
Medial Plating Studies	Cohen D	Medial Plate	Postoperative Ulnar Neuritis	P Value
Wiggers et al,[16] 2012	0.597	107	14	.02
Ilyas	0.863	21	8	.051
	Weighted effect size (Cohen D) 0.64			

the control group (no medial plate) based on a probability of superiority. In order to have one more unfavorable outcome in the treatment group compared with the control group, 5 patients would need to be treated; if 100 people go through the procedure with medial plating, 21 more people will have ulnar neuropathy with a medial plate as compared with the control group.

DISCUSSION

Despite advances in the management of distal humerus fractures, complications, such as ulnar neuropathy, continue to pose a challenge. The development of ulnar neuropathy has many potential causes. The ulnar nerve may be contused or lacerated at the time of the initial trauma. Iatrogenic causes of ulnar nerve injury include excessive retraction or inadvertent injury during surgical exposure, fracture manipulation, or hardware placement. Surgeon-related technical causes of a postoperative ulnar nerve injury, whether managed in situ or transposed, can include inadequate decompression, aggressive decompression with devascularization of the nerve, or traumatic handling of the nerve during its dissection. Similarly, swelling and hematoma formation in the immediate perioperative period may also contribute to injury to the ulnar nerve. Delayed causes of ulnar neuropathy can be related to limitations in motion and in particular loss of

terminal extension, soft tissue scarring, heterotopic ossification, and prominent hardware. As evidenced from the earlier discussion, the ulnar nerve is at risk preoperatively at the time of the injury, intraoperatively during exposure and fixation, and even postoperatively during healing. Although most studies report the incidence of ulnar neuropathy between 0% and 38%, one study reported a rate of 51%.[7] Because of this high prevalence, careful planning and management of the ulnar nerve is necessary. Unfortunately, no prospective cohort studies or randomized trials exist that reliably and objectively diagnose preoperative ulnar nerve dysfunction, immediate postoperative function, and delayed postoperative ulnar nerve dysfunction. Moreover, the surgical handling of the ulnar nerve has also not been standardized and is often not well documented in published series.

The findings of this meta-analysis yield that in situ management of the ulnar nerve resulted in less postoperative ulnar neuropathy than with transposition. The potential advantages and disadvantages of in situ management of the ulnar nerve are less nerve manipulation and compromised vascularity but more risk of direct nerve injury during fracture fixation. In contrast, the potential advantages and disadvantages of transposition are greater nerve protection by moving it away from the fracture site but with more risk of nerve injury, devascularization, and scar formation following greater nerve manipulation. Overall, the authors found the overall incidence of ulnar neuropathy of 19.3% reasonable but were surprised that transposition resulted in greater postoperative neuropathy than in situ management. This surprise was based on 2 assumptions: first, that equality exists between in situ decompression and transposition in primary nontraumatic ulnar neuropathy of the elbow[17] and, second, that a transposition would minimize direct nerve injury during fracture manipulation perioperatively and that transposition would protect better against swelling and prolonged flexion postoperatively.

Regarding the fixation strategy, often medial and lateral plates are needed to manage distal humerus fractures. Based on the authors' data using weighted effect sizes (see **Table 2**), more patients will have postoperative ulnar neuropathy with a medial plate. They found this result to be intuitive, as the plate would likely require more manipulation of the nerve intraoperatively and could potentially cause irritation and perineural scarring postoperatively. Ultimately, the decision to apply a plate medially will be based on the needs of adequate fracture fixation. However, the findings of this meta-analysis can be considered to avoid medial plating, if not absolutely necessary for fracture fixation.

This meta-analysis, like most, has several shortcomings. The primary limitation is the heterogeneity of the included retrospective studies as well as the deficiency in the number of studies. Specific to this meta-analysis, preexisting ulnar nerve dysfunction is not clearly defined in all of these studies nor is the total recovery time from ulnar nerve injury. Furthermore, the degree of injury that the ulnar nerve suffered in each case is not clear, as it was not reliably classified in a consistent manner. Lastly, the surgeon's rationale of choosing either in situ management or transposition was no well documented and the surgical technique that was used was not always well described.

SUMMARY

There is a substantial incidence of postoperative ulnar nerve dysfunction following open reduction and plate and screw fixation of the distal humerus. The goal of this meta-analysis was to assess if a best method exists for handling the ulnar nerve, specifically whether in situ decompression versus ulnar nerve transposition results in a lower incidence of postoperative ulnar neuropathy. A secondary goal was to assess if the plate position contributed to nerve dysfunction. The authors found that postoperative ulnar neuropathy was more prevalent in those patients who underwent a transposition as opposed to in situ management. The authors can

draw the conclusion that transposition of the ulnar nerve during this procedure does not have a protective effect, and instead in situ release may be more advantageous. Moreover, the findings of this meta-analysis discourage the placement of a medial plate when mechanically allowed.

REFERENCES

1. Galano GJ, Ahmad CS, Levine WN. Current treatment strategies for bicolumnar distal humerus fractures. J Am Acad Orthop Surg 2010;18(1):20–30.
2. Zlotolow DA, Catalano LW III, Barron OA, et al. Surgical exposures of the humerus. J Am Acad Orthop Surg 2006;14:754–65.
3. McKee M, Veillette CJ, Hall JA, et al. A multicenter, prospective, randomized, controlled trial of open reduction-internal fixation versus total elbow arthroplasty for displaced intra-articular distal humeral fractures in elderly patients. J Shoulder Elbow Surg 2009;18:3–12.
4. Ring D, Jupiter JB. Complex fractures of the distal humerus and their complications. J Shoulder Elbow Surg 1999;8:85–97.
5. Sodergard J, Sandelin J, Bostman O. Postoperative complications of distal humerus fractures. Acta Orthop Scand 1992;63(1):85–9.
6. Gofton WT, Macdermid JC, Patterson SD, et al. Functional outcome of AO type C distal humeral fractures. J Hand Surg Am 2003;28(2):294–308.
7. Holdsworth BJ, Mossad MM. Fractures of the adult distal humerus. Elbow function after internal fixation. J Bone Joint Surg Br 1990;72(3):362–5.
8. Huang JI, Paczas M, Hoyen HA, et al. Functional outcome after open reduction internal fixation of intra-articular fractures of the distal humerus in the elderly. J Orthop Trauma 2011;25(5):259–65.
9. Doornberg JN, van Duijn PJ, Linzel D, et al. Surgical treatment of intra-articular fractures of the distal part of the humerus. Functional outcome after twelve to thirty years. J Bone Joint Surg Am 2007;89(7):1524–32.
10. Vazquez O, Rutgers M, Ring DC, et al. Fate of the ulnar nerve after operative fixation of distal humerus fractures. J Orthop Trauma 2010;24(7):395–9.
11. Chen RC, Harris DJ, Leduc S, et al. Is ulnar nerve transposition beneficial during open reduction internal fixation of distal humerus fractures? J Orthop Trauma 2010;24(7):391–4.
12. Ruan HJ, Liu JJ, Fan CY, et al. Incidence, management, and prognosis of early nerve dysfunction in type C fractures of distal humerus. J Orthop Trauma 2009;67(6):1397–401.
13. Worden A, Ilyas AM. Ulnar neuropathy following distal humerus fracture fixation. Orthop Clin North Am 2012;43(4):509–14.
14. McGowan A. The results of transposition of the ulnar nerve for traumatic ulnar neuritis. J Bone Joint Surg Br 1950;32-B(3):293–301.

15. Wang KC, Shih HN, Hsu KY, et al. Intercondylar fractures of the distal humerus: routine anterior subcutaneous transposition of the ulnar nerve in a posterior operative approach. J Orthop Trauma 1994;36(6):770–3.

16. Wiggers JK, Brouwer KM, Helmerhorst GTT, et al. Predictors of diagnosis of ulnar neuropathy after surgically treated distal humerus fractures. J Hand Surg Am 2012;37(6):1168–72.

17. Macadam SA, Gandhi R, Bezuhly M, et al. Simple decompression versus anterior subcutaneous and submuscular transposition of the ulnar nerve for cubital tunnel syndrome: a meta-analysis. J Hand Surg Am 2008;33A:1314–24.

Radial Nerve Palsy After Humeral Shaft Fractures
The Case for Early Exploration and a New Classification to Guide Treatment and Prognosis

Gerard Chang, MD*, Asif M. Ilyas, MD

KEYWORDS

- Radial nerve palsy • Humerus fracture • Holstein-Lewis fracture

KEY POINTS

- Radial nerve palsies are common peripheral nerve palsies associated with 2% to 17% of humeral shaft fractures.
- Primary radial nerve palsies associated with closed humeral shaft fractures have a recovery rate in 70% to 88% of cases.
- Radial nerve palsies with humerus fractures can be classified as type 1 neuropraxia, type 2 incarcerated, type 3 partial transection, and type 4 complete transection.
- Surgical exploration is recommended for radial nerve palsies associated with open fractures, fractures that cannot achieve an adequate closed reduction requiring fracture repair, fractures with associated vascular injuries, and polytrauma patients.
- Early exploration in all cases can potentially expedite nerve injury characterization and treatment if it is lacerated or incarcerated and facilitates early fracture stabilization and quicker rehabilitation, while also minimizing nerve end plate loss and muscular atrophy and decreasing loss of time and livelihood for patients associated with delayed exploration in cases without spontaneous nerve recovery.

INTRODUCTION

Fractures of the humeral shaft are common injuries managed by orthopedic surgeons. In the United States, more than 237,000 humerus fractures occur each year, representing between 1% and 5% of all fractures.[1,2] Retrospective studies have demonstrated that these fractures follow a bimodal distribution occurring most commonly in younger men with high-energy trauma and older women involved in low-energy trauma, such as falls from standing.[3–5] In a large systematic review, transverse and spiral fracture patterns of the humeral shaft were found to be more common than oblique and complex comminuted fracture patterns.[6]

Complicating humerus fractures are injuries to the surrounding nerves. Damage to the radial nerve in humeral shaft fractures is the most common nerve lesion complicating fractures of long bones.[6] The nature of the radial nerve palsy itself is variable and can range from a transient contusion or neuropraxia to nerve incarceration between fracture fragments, partial laceration, and even complete transection (**Fig. 1**). The authors propose a new classification of radial nerve palsies

Rothman Institute at Thomas Jefferson University, 925 Chestnut Street, Philadelphia, PA 19107, USA
* Corresponding author. Thomas Jefferson University Hospital, 111 South 11th Street, Philadelphia, PA 19107.
E-mail address: gerard.chang@gmail.com

Hand Clin 34 (2018) 105–112
https://doi.org/10.1016/j.hcl.2017.09.011
0749-0712/18/© 2017 Elsevier Inc. All rights reserved.

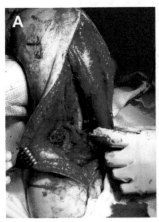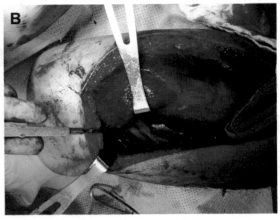

Fig. 1. Two cases of radial nerve palsy occurring primarily with spiral fractures of the humerus repaired with a posterior approach through a lateral para-tricipital window: (*A*) An incarcerated nerve found sitting within the fracture site. (*B*) A partially lacerated nerve found draped over the sharp end of the fracture.

to guide treatment and prognosis based on intraoperative findings on exploration (**Table 1**).

Studies have shown the incidence of radial nerve palsy associated with humeral shaft fractures to be anywhere between 2% and 17%.[6–9] In a systematic review of 1045 cases of humeral shaft fractures, Shao and colleagues[6] identified an incidence of radial nerve palsy to be 11.8%, with spontaneous recovery occurring in 70.7% of cases without surgical exploration. The recovery rate increased to 88.1% when cases of both early and late surgical exploration were included.

ANATOMY

The course of the radial nerve through the posterior compartment of the arm has classically been described as following between the origins of the medial and lateral heads of the triceps, lying intimately along the cortex of spiral groove, placing it

Table 1
New classification system of radial nerve palsies to guide treatment and prognosis based on intraoperative findings on exploration

New Classification	Treatment
Type 1: Stretch/ neuropraxia	Neurolysis
Type 2: Incarcerated	Extrication of the nerve
Type 3: Partial transection	Repair of the nerve, with possible wrapping
Type 4: Complete transection	Repair of the nerve, with possible grafting

at increased risk for damage from humeral shaft fractures. However, the spiral groove is the origin of the brachialis muscle and it, along with the origin muscle fibers of the medial head of the triceps, separate the radial nerve from the cortex along most of the musculospiral groove. Distally, as the nerve approaches the lateral intermuscular septum and lateral condylar ridge, the nerve does contact the lower margin of the spiral groove for variable distances, anywhere between 0 and 7 cm, depending on the thickness of the muscle deep to the nerve, with the thicker specimens resulting in less contact.[7,10] Fractures of the humerus can be classified by their anatomic location, separating the humeral shaft into thirds. Holstein and Lewis[7] described an association between radial nerve injury and spiral fractures of the distal third humeral shaft, which has since been referred to as a Holstein-Lewis fracture. (**Fig. 2**) Their proposed mechanism of injury is when the spiral fracture occurs, the proximal segment advances distally, which displaces the lateral intermuscular septum that the radial nerve runs through and, therefore, puts it at risk of getting tethered and injured. Another proposed mechanism is when the distal segment moves proximally and laterally, the apex of the fragment can lacerate the nerve. A cadaveric study by Carlan and colleagues[11] found the radial nerve to be at risk of injury with fractures of the humerus in 2 regions: posterior midshaft area at the distal aspect of the deltoid tuberosity and along the lateral distal third aspect of the humerus approximately 11 cm proximal to the lateral epicondyle. Reports of the incidence of radial nerve injury based on anatomic location of the fracture has been mixed. Bostman and colleagues[12] found an equal incidence of radial nerve palsies in fractures of the middle and distal third of the humeral shaft.

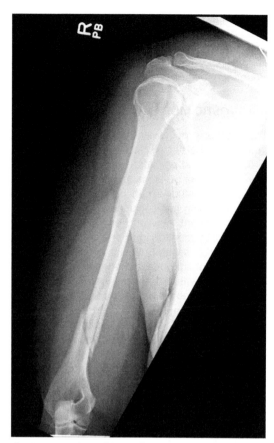

Fig. 2. A spiral or oblique fracture of the distal third of the humeral shaft classically associated with radial nerve palsies. However, radial nerve palsies are not exclusively associated with this pattern.

However, one report noted a higher likelihood of radial nerve injury in middle third fractures,[8] whereas others have found an increased incidence of radial nerve injury in fractures of the distal third.[13]

DIAGNOSIS

Every evaluation of a humeral shaft fracture begins with a thorough physical examination, consisting of sensory and motor evaluation of the median, ulnar, and radial nerves. Specifically, radial nerve sensation can be tested to light touch and pinprick on the dorsum of the hand over the first web space. Radial nerve motor function can be evaluated with active extension of the wrist and of the fingers at the metacarpophalangeal joints. Testing for the absence of brachioradialis or extensor carpi radialis longus firing may provide additional information indicating a more proximal injury at the level of the humeral shaft.[14]

CLASSIFICATION

There are several ways to classify a radial nerve palsy associated with a humeral shaft fracture:

complete or partial, primary versus secondary, Seddon or Sunderland types, or a new classification proposed in this report that could better guide treatment and prognosis.

Complete palsies, meaning no motor function or sensation, have been reported to occur in 50% to 68% of radial nerve palsies.[8,13] Peripheral nerve injuries can be further characterized by the classification system developed by Seddon[15] in 1942. He described 3 basic types of nerve injury: neurapraxia, axonotmesis, and neurotmesis. Eight years later, Sunderland[16] expanded Seddon's classification to further separate degrees of neurotmesis based on the severity of injury.[15]

Primary nerve palsies happen at the time of injury and are discovered on the initial assessment. These palsies typically arise after closed management with or without manipulation and even after surgical treatment. Most secondary radial nerve palsies arise from closed management with or without manipulation of the humerus fracture.[17] Previous reports have cited secondary radial nerve palsies as an absolute indication for exploration.[13,17,18] However, more recent studies have shown convincing evidence that secondary palsies can be treated similar to its primary counterparts.[6,12,17,19]

Secondary palsies can occur anytime during treatment after a documented initial intact examination. Surgical management of humeral shaft fractures is a common cause of secondary nerve palsies. The least invasive surgical treatment option is with intramedullary nailing; however, this is not recommended in primary radial nerve palsies associated with humeral shaft fractures because of the potential for entrapment of the nerve in the fracture site leaving it vulnerable to further damage during canal preparation and rod insertion. The incidence of secondary palsies following intramedullary nailing has been reported to be somewhere between 0% and 5%.[20] However, several studies have shown these secondary palsies to be temporary and resolve spontaneously.[21–24] According to the literature, the incidence of secondary radial nerve palsies after open reduction internal fixation with compression plating is up to 10%.[25,26] This technique offers the ability for direct visualization and anatomic reduction as well as provides the most predictable union rate. In addition, it allows for exploration of the radial nerve. Routine exploration of the entire radial nerve is advised during open reduction internal fixation, especially for patients with primary nerve palsies. Even for patients without nerve palsies, it is recommended to explore the nerve, tag it, and ensure the plate sits underneath the nerve to avoid iatrogenic entrapment (**Fig. 3**). One study of secondary radial

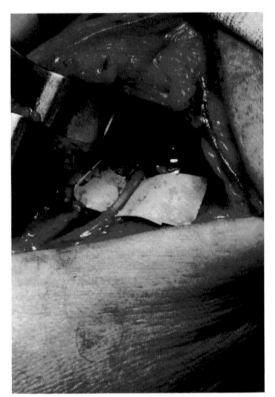

Fig. 3. Iatrogenic entrapment of the radial nerve followed by plating of the humeral shaft through an anterolateral approach. The radial nerve injury was found with re-exploration after failure of spontaneous recovery of a secondary nerve palsy.

nerve palsies following surgical management found them to be significantly more common (41 of 47) following open reduction internal fixation; however, they showed a high rate of spontaneous recovery and shorter recovery time compared with primary palsies.[19]

The new classification being proposed is based on the assessment of the radial nerve on exploration (see **Table 1**). It is anticipated that a type 1 injury, neuropraxia, would recover spontaneously and requires no further treatment other than fracture fixation while protecting the nerve from surgical iatrogenic injury. Type 2 injuries (see **Fig. 1**A) represent a unique circumstance whereby the nerve is most likely suffering from neuropraxia but is also incarcerated between fracture fragments, thereby making it vulnerable to being incarcerated and compressed within the fracture callus. Type 3 (partial transection) nerve injuries can be treated with direct nerve repair. Similarly, type 4 (complete transection) nerve injuries can be treated with direct nerve repair or with a nerve graft if the extent of retraction and/or the gap following nerve ending debridement prohibits direct nerve

repair. In all cases with nerve exploration, internal fixation of the humerus is also recommended to encourage primary bone healing and avoid secondary injury to the nerve with callus formation (secondary bone healing) and macro-motion.

DIAGNOSTIC MODALITIES

The diagnosis of humeral shaft fractures with a radial nerve palsy can readily be made with plain radiographs and physical examination. However, there is a role for other diagnostic modalities. Electrodiagnostic studies can be particularly helpful when evaluating nerve injuries by determining the level and extent of injury, establishing baseline function, and monitoring improvement. However, in the initial several weeks, electrodiagnostic studies are of little benefit because these studies cannot differentiate between nerve injuries that will or will not recover spontaneously.[14] For those managing these injuries with observation, an electrodiagnostic study at 3 weeks or later is better for establishing baseline function by showing fibrillation potentials, positive sharp waves, and monophasic action potentials of short duration.[27] In addition, an electrodiagnostic study at this point can show indicators of prognosis. In one study looking at prognostic electrodiagnostic markers in traumatic radial nerve palsies, recruitment of brachioradialis and compound muscle action potential amplitude measured from the extensor indices proved to be the best indicators for good outcomes.[28] If the nerve palsy persists with no clinical improvement beyond 8 weeks, another electrodiagnostic study may be helpful.[29] In one series, all patients who spontaneously regained function after a radial nerve palsy associated with humeral shaft fractures showed clinical signs of improvement within the first 2 months.[17] By 12 weeks, motor unit potentials should be present on electromyography and can help distinguish injuries that will spontaneously recover and those that will not.[14] In addition, if the study shows improvement from the baseline study with larger polyphasic motor unit action potentials of longer duration, then one can expect further spontaneous recovery to occur.[27] However, if there is no improvement at 12 weeks from the baseline study, exploration may be warranted.

Other imaging modalities, specifically ultrasound and MRI, are presently being researched and show a promising ability to assist in characterizing these injuries. However, there is not enough clinical evidence to warrant their routine use at this time. Bodner and colleagues[30] showed they were able to differentiate severely damaged radial nerves (confirmed intraoperatively) from those with minor damage, which all recovered spontaneously, using ultrasound. Recently, much research has been conducted looking at the role of MRI in traumatic peripheral nerve injury in determining the degree of injury and prognosis. Deniel and colleagues[31] suggested that the Seddon classification of nerve injury could be determined within the first 48 hours of injury using MRI. Furthermore, Simon and colleagues[32] discussed the ability of diffusion-tensor MRI to show the evolutionary changes of degeneration verses regeneration following nerve injury, which may allow for the important distinction between axonotmetic and neurotmetic injury.

TREATMENT STRATEGIES

Despite numerous studies, the management of radial nerve palsies associated with humeral shaft fractures remains a controversial topic. There are a few circumstances in which there is little controversy, and early exploration is the well-accepted standard of care. These circumstances include open fractures, fractures that cannot achieve an adequate closed reduction and require open reduction internal fixation, fractures with associated vascular injuries, and polytrauma patients.[7–9,13,25,33–35] Palsies associated with gunshot fractures of the humerus are unique scenarios that, according to Bercik and colleagues,[36] can be managed expectantly unless associated with concomitant vascular injury. Earlier reports included secondary palsies after closed reduction as an absolute indication; however, as cited earlier, there is growing evidence that these too can be managed expectantly. For the typical primary radial nerve palsy associated with a closed humeral shaft fracture, in general, the debate is split between 2 basic camps of thought: practitioners favoring early exploration versus those favoring expectant management with possible late exploration.

Early Exploration

Proponents of early exploration in all cases with a radial nerve palsy with a humerus fracture argue that all radial nerve palsies following humeral shaft fractures should be treated with early exploration.[13,34,37] They support this position by claiming the following advantages.

- Early exploration is indicated, as a sufficient number of radial nerve palsies do not recover spontaneously (approximately 30% of cases[6]), thereby still warranting late exploration 3 months after injury prolonging

rehabilitation, disability, and potentially compromising nerve recovery.
- Early exploration allows for early nerve injury characterization and classification (neuropraxia, incarceration, partial transection, and complete transection) and subsequent early treatment and recovery before the setting-in of soft tissue scarring, nerve retraction, motor end plate loss, and muscular atrophy.
- Early exploration and nerve repair (if incarcerated or transected) leads to superior outcomes, as nerve recovery outcomes are time dependent.
- Early exploration is technically easier and safer than late exploration, with the latter being more prone to soft tissue scarring and potential entrapment of the nerve in fracture callus.
- Early nerve exploration affords concomitant fracture stabilization with internal fixation, thereby facilitating quicker functional recovery and rehabilitation of patients.
- Early exploration and fracture repair facilitates primary bone healing and decreases the chances of secondary bone healing and entrapment or compression of the nerve in fracture callus.

According to some investigators, there are too many radial nerve injuries that require surgical treatment to not exercise early exploration in all palsies associated with fractures. Depending on the series reported, the proportion of surgically treatable lesions following late exploration varies. In a series by Foster and colleagues[35] of humeral shaft fractures treated openly, 9 of 14 were found to have radial nerve laceration or entrapment requiring surgical treatment. The true number of surgically correctable lesions likely falls between 6% and 25%.[8,34,38–41] Kaiser and company[37] stated, "Remedial lesions were encountered too frequently to ignore early exploration."

The next argument points to the fact that earlier nerve repair leads to superior outcomes. According to Sunderland,[42] a delay of more than 12 months does not worsen outcomes. However, Seddon[43] states that a good prognosis is more likely if it is treated before 12 months. Lowe and colleagues[14] supports this stand, affirming that the timing of nerve repair is paramount and that motor end plates must be reinnervated by 12 months for useful function to be restored; however, irrecoverable muscle atrophy can ensue sooner.[14] There is further evidence in the literature to support that delays beyond even 5 months have shown inferior outcomes.[9] Advocates of early exploration also claim it is technically easier, safer, and reduces the chance that the radial nerve remains enveloped in callus and scar tissue. A case report from Ikeda and Osamura[44] shows how challenging a nerve repair can be when enveloped in fracture callus. In this specific case, the nerve could not be safely released from the fracture callus and was, therefore, sharply dissected at the bone and repaired end to end.

In short, delayed exploration and observation of patients with a lacerated or incarcerated radial nerve will result in a lack of early functional recovery, potential muscle atrophy and motor end plate loss, and substantial interim loss of patient function and livelihood. On the other hand, early exploration and repair can expedite quicker characterization of the nerve injury, quicker return of function, and, most importantly to some, peace of mind. Furthermore, on stabilization of the fracture with open reduction internal fixation, a repaired nerve will theoretically benefit from a better environment for healing with less traction, motion, or callus formation to impede nerve regeneration.

Observation/Delayed Exploration

Although early investigators recommended routine surgical exploration of all radial nerve palsies associated with humeral shaft fractures, with time, the pendulum has shifted and investigators have begun favoring no immediate treatment because of a high rate of recovery, more than 70%.[3,13,25,34,38,39] In a systematic review conducted by Shao and colleagues[6] of primary radial nerve palsies associated with humerus fractures, they found a spontaneous recovery rate of 70.7% and an overall recovery rate of 88.1%. In addition, they did not find any difference in outcomes between patients managed with early exploration and observation.[6] This finding was later confirmed in a meta-analysis by Liu and company.[45] In light of a high recovery rate and equal outcomes, advocates in this camp claim many unnecessary surgical procedures, along with their risks, can be avoided with initial the observation.

In short, proponents of delayed exploration argue that many of the standard risks associated with surgery, such as pain, bleeding, infection, and scarring, can be avoided in patients whom may otherwise recover with full function without any surgical intervention.

In regard to timing of delayed exploration, the literature also varies. Shaw and Sakellarides[38] concluded from their series that because all patients who spontaneously recovered full motor function showed signs of recovery within the first 2 months, any patient who does not show any evidence of recovery by 8 weeks should be explored. Goldner and Kelley[46] supported this

recommendation, even though in their series some patients who recovered completely did not show any signs of recovery within the first 20 weeks. Amillo and company,[9] based on their findings, endorsed exploration at 3 months if there were no clinical or electrophysiologic signs of recovery.

SUMMARY

Radial nerve palsies are relatively frequent complications associated with humeral shaft fractures, with an incidence of 2% to 17%. These injuries can be classified as either partial or complete, depending on the degree of injury, and primary or secondary, depending on the timing of the palsy's presentation. The authors have proposed a classification based on the intraoperative condition of the nerve with type 1 representing neuropraxia, type 2 nerve incarceration within fracture fragments or comminution, type 3 a partial transection, and type 4 a complete transection.

Early exploration is recommended for open fractures, fractures that cannot achieve an adequate closed reduction and require open reduction internal fixation, fractures with associated vascular injuries, and polytrauma patients. Initial management of radial nerve palsies associated with closed fractures of the humerus still remains a controversial topic. Traditional recommendations were observation with late exploration limited to cases without spontaneous nerve recovery at 3 to 6 months. In doing so, many patients could avoid unnecessary surgeries and the complications associated with them because these injuries have historically had a high spontaneous recovery rate. Proponents of early exploration think that the initial observation for spontaneous recovery with delayed exploration if necessary can lead to increased muscular atrophy, motor end plate loss, nerve entrapment in fracture callus, compromised nerve recovery on delayed repair, and significant interval loss of patient function and livelihood. On the other hand, early exploration allows for prompt nerve injury characterization and treatment and enables early fracture stabilization, which can prevent late nerve injury or incarceration, and, most importantly for some, peace of mind. Furthermore, early exploration revealing a nerve injury that can be repaired can lead to quicker nerve recovery with less motor end plate loss, less muscular atrophy, and a quicker return to function.

REFERENCES

1. Ward EF, Savoie FH, Hughes JL. Fractures of the diaphyseal humerus. In: Browner BD, Jupiter JB, Levine AM, et al, editors. Skeletal trauma. 2nd edition. Philadelphia: WB Saunders Co; 1998. p. 1523–47.

2. Ekholm R, Adami J, Tidermark J, et al. Fractures of the shaft of the humerus. An epidemiological study of 401 fractures. J Bone Joint Surg Br 2006;88(11): 1469–73.

3. Mast JW, Spiegel PG, Harvey JPJ, et al. Fractures of the humeral shaft: a retrospective study of 240 adult fractures. Clin Orthop Relat Res 1975;112:254–62.

4. Rose SH, Melton LJ III, Morrey BF, et al. Epidemiologic features of humeral fractures. Clin Orthop Relat Res 1982;168:24–30.

5. Tytherleigh-Strong G, Walls N, McQueen MM. The epidemiology of humeral shaft fractures. J Bone Joint Surg Br 1998;80(2):249–53.

6. Shao YC, Harwood P, Grotz MRW, et al. Radial nerve palsy associated with fractures of the shaft of the humerus: a systematic review. J Bone Joint Surg Br 2005;87(12):1647–52.

7. Holstein A, Lewis GM. Fractures of the humerus with radial-nerve paralysis. J Bone Joint Surg Am 1963; 45:1382–8.

8. Pollock FH, Drake D, Bovill EG, et al. Treatment of radial neuropathy associated with fractures of the humerus. J Bone Joint Surg Am 1981;63(2):239–43.

9. Amillo S, Barrios RH, Martínez-Peric R, et al. Surgical treatment of the radial nerve lesions associated with fractures of the humerus. J Orthop Trauma 1993;7(3):211–5.

10. Whitson RO. Relation of the radial nerve to the shaft of the humerus. J Bone Joint Surg Am 1954;36-A(1): 85–8.

11. Carlan D, Pratt J, Patterson JMM, et al. The radial nerve in the brachium: an anatomic study in human cadavers. J Hand Surg 2007;32(8):1177–82.

12. Bostman O, Bakalim G, Vainionpaa S, et al. Radial palsy in shaft fracture of the humerus. Acta Orthop Scand 1986;57(4):316–9.

13. Garcia AJ, Maeck BH. Radial nerve injuries in fractures of the shaft of the humerus. Am J Surg 1960; 99:625–7.

14. Lowe JB 3rd, Sen SK, Mackinnon SE. Current approach to radial nerve paralysis. Plast Reconstr Surg 2002;110(4):1099–113.

15. Seddon HJ. A classification of nerve injuries. Br Med J 1942;2(4260):237–9.

16. Sunderland S. A classification of peripheral nerve injuries producing loss of function. Brain 1951;74(4): 491–516.

17. Shah JJ, Bhatti NA. Radial nerve paralysis associated with fractures of the humerus. A review of 62 cases. Clin Orthop Relat Res 1983;172:171–6.

18. Duncan DM, Johnson KA, Monkman GR. Fracture of the humerus and radial nerve palsy. Minn Med 1974; 57(8):659–62.

19. Lang NW, Ostermann RC, Arthold C, et al. Retrospective case series with one year follow-up after radial nerve palsy associated with humeral fractures. Int Orthop 2017;41(1):191–6.

20. Farragos AF, Schemitsch EH, McKee MD. Complications of intramedullary nailing for fractures of the humeral shaft: a review. J Orthop Trauma 1999;13(4): 258–67.

21. Crolla RM, de Vries LS, Clevers GJ. Locked intramedullary nailing of humeral fractures. Injury 1993; 24(6):403–6.

22. Rommens PM, Verbruggen J, Broos PL. Retrograde locked nailing of humeral shaft fractures. A review of 39 patients. J Bone Joint Surg Br 1995;77(1): 84–9.

23. Ingman AM, Waters DA. Locked intramedullary nailing of humeral shaft fractures. Implant design, surgical technique, and clinical results. J Bone Joint Surg Br 1994;76(1):23–9.

24. Ajmal M, O'Sullivan M, McCabe J, et al. Antegrade locked intramedullary nailing in humeral shaft fractures. Injury 2001;32(9):692–4.

25. Dabezies EJ, Banta CJ 2nd, Murphy CP, et al. Plate fixation of the humeral shaft for acute fractures, with and without radial nerve injuries. J Orthop Trauma 1992;6(1):10–3.

26. Bell MJ, Beauchamp CG, Kellam JK, et al. The results of plating humeral shaft fractures in patients with multiple injuries. The Sunnybrook experience. J Bone Joint Surg Br 1985;67(2):293–6.

27. Mohler LR, Hanel DP. Closed fractures complicated by peripheral nerve injury. J Am Acad Orthop Surg 2006;14(1):32–7.

28. Malikowski T, Micklesen PJ, Robinson LR. Prognostic values of electrodiagnostic studies in traumatic radial neuropathy. Muscle Nerve 2007;36(3): 364–7.

29. Robinson LR. traumatic injury to peripheral nerves. Suppl Clin Neurophysiol 2004;57:173–86.

30. Bodner G, Buchberger W, Schocke M, et al. Radial nerve palsy associated with humeral shaft fracture: evaluation with US–initial experience. Radiology 2001;219(3):811–6.

31. Deniel A, Causeret A, Moser T, et al. Entrapment and traumatic neuropathies of the elbow and hand: an imaging approach. Diagn Interv Imaging 2015; 96(12):1261–78.

32. Simon NG, Narvid J, Cage T, et al. Visualizing axon regeneration after peripheral nerve injury with magnetic resonance tractography. Neurology 2014; 83(15):1382–4.

33. Heim D, Herkert F, Hess P, et al. Surgical treatment of humeral shaft fractures–the Basel experience. J Trauma 1993;35(2):226–32.

34. Packer JW, Foster RR, Garcia A, et al. The humeral fracture with radial nerve palsy: is exploration warranted? Clin Orthop Relat Res 1972;88: 34–8.

35. Foster RJ, Swiontkowski MF, Bach AW, et al. Radial nerve palsy caused by open humeral shaft fractures. J Hand Surg Am 1993;18(1):121–4.

36. Bercik MJ, Kingsbery J, Ilyas AM. Peripheral nerve injuries following gunshot fracture of the humerus. Orthopedics 2012;35(3):e349–52.

37. Kaiser TE, Sim FH, Kelly PJ. Radial nerve palsy associated with humeral fractures. Orthopedics 1981;4(11):1245–51.

38. Shaw JL, Sakellarides H. Radial-nerve paralysis associated with fractures of the humerus. A review of forty-five cases. J Bone Joint Surg Am 1967; 49(5):899–902.

39. Kettelkamp DB, Alexander H. Clinical review of radial nerve injury. J Trauma 1967;7(3):424–32.

40. Klenerman L. Fractures of the shaft of the humerus. J Bone Joint Surg Br 1966;48(1):105–11.

41. Seddon HJ. Nerve lesions complicating certain closed bone injuries. JAMA 1947;135(11):691–4.

42. Sunderland S. When are attempts at nerve repair no longer justified?. In: Sunderland S, editor. Nerves and nerve injuries. Edinburgh (United Kingdom): Churchill Livingstone; 1978. p. 507–9.

43. Seddon H. Factors influencing indications for operation. In: Seddon H, editor. Surgical disorders of the peripheral nerves. Baltimore (MD): Williams & Wilkins; 1972. p. 240–5.

44. Ikeda K, Osamura N. The radial nerve palsy caused by embedding in the humeral shaft fracture - a case report. Hand Surg 2014;19(1):91–3.

45. Liu G, Zhang C, Wu H. Comparison of initial nonoperative and operative management of radial nerve palsy associated with acute humeral shaft fractures. Orthopedics 2012;35(8):702–8.

46. Goldner J, Kelley JM. Radial nerve injuries. South Med J 1958;51:873–83.

Distal Radius Fractures in a Functional Quadruped

Spanning Bridge Plate Fixation of the Wrist

Brian A. Tinsley, MD, Asif M. Ilyas, MD*

CrossMark

KEYWORDS

- Distal radius fractures • Functional quadruped • Spanning bridge plate fixation • Wrist

KEY POINTS

- Functional quadrupeds are patients who require full weight bearing with all 4 extremities in order to mobilize and bear weight.
- A functional quadruped can be someone who is walker dependent to mobilize or patients with polytrauma temporarily needing their upper extremities to bear weight and mobilize with crutches or a walker.
- In a functional quadruped, distal radius fractures can be treated with a dorsal spanning bridge plate for any fracture pattern to allow immediate unrestricted weight bearing with the injured upper extremity.
- In the authors' series, there were no cases of nonunions, tendon ruptures, or reoperations other than the planned staged bridge plate removal.
- Dorsal spanning bridge plate fixation of distal radius fractures in the functional quadruped is a viable treatment strategy for immediate weight bearing with the injured limb and, in the authors' series, demonstrates satisfactory results.

INTRODUCTION

The prevalence of distal radius fractures continues to increase as the average age of the US population increases.[1] Among patients more than 65 years of age, distal radius fractures account for 18% of all fractures.[2] Although there is an increasing trend toward treating distal radial fractures operatively, elderly patients are better able to tolerate malunion compared with younger patients relative to ultimate functional outcomes.[3–5] The treatment of distal radius fractures includes nonoperative treatment with splint or cast immobilization as well as multiple operative options with surgical fixation. Broadly, the indications for surgical fixation of a distal radius fracture include unstable and/or displaced fractures. However, additional surgical indications for distal radius fractures include polytrauma patients and walker-dependent elderly patients, both needing the use of their hands for weight bearing and mobilization, that is, a *functional quadruped*. A quadruped is an animal with 4 feet, and humans are, by definition, biped. However, patients with lower-extremity injuries and/or patients who normally depend on assistive devices, such as a walker, are essentially a functional quadruped, as they require all 4 limbs in order to mobilize and ambulate.

A functional quadruped with a distal radius fracture, irrespective of fracture pattern specifics,

Ethical Board Review Statement: No animals or human subjects.

Conflict of Interest Statement: An author of this study (A.M.I.) serves as design surgeon and paid consultant for Globus (Audobon, PA, USA).

Rothman Institute at Thomas Jefferson University, 925 Chestnut Street, Philadelphia, PA 19107, USA

* Corresponding author.

E-mail address: asif.ilyas@rothmaninstitute.com

hand.theclinics.com

poses a unique challenge. Standard surgical fixation options of the distal radius include closed reduction and pinning with casting, external fixation, fragment-specific fixation, intramedullary nailing, and various plating options, including volar, dorsal, and radial plates.[6] However, except for external fixation, the other surgical options for the distal radius do not necessarily afford immediate weight bearing with an assistive device like a cane, crutch, or walker. In these settings, an alternative surgical fixation option is the use of a spanning dorsal bridge plate.[7,8]

The concept of dorsal spanning or bridge plate fixation of distal radius fractures is not new and was initially described to manage either highly comminuted fractures of the distal radius and/or serve as an alternative to cases requiring prolonged external fixation as an internal fixator instead.[7,9] This technique has evolved, and its indications have expanded to include polytrauma patients with the particular goal of earlier weight bearing with the injured upper extremity and improved rehabilitation.[10] The traditional technique used an Association for Osteosynthesis (AO)/Association for the Study of Internal Fixation's 3.5-mm dynamic compression plate (DCP) applied in a noncompression fashion (**Fig. 1**). More recently, contoured low-profile locking plates have become available, increasing its ease

of application and the application in functional quadruped patients with a distal radius fracture (**Fig. 2**).[8]

INDICATIONS AND CONTRAINDICATIONS

The relative indication for a dorsal spanning bridge plate fixation of a distal radial fracture includes any patient with a distal radius fracture who is a functional quadruped requiring full weight bearing on the injured extremity in order to ambulate with an assistive device. In these patients, the goal is immediate unrestricted weight bearing; thus, any distal radius fracture is indicated. Additional treatment options specific to the use of a dorsal spanning bridge plate include complex articular fractures and/or fractures with significant meta-diaphyseal comminution or bone loss.[7,8] Contraindications include patients with large open dorsal wounds that would result in exposed hardware.

TECHNIQUE

Either a small-fragment 3.5-mm locking DCP or a commercially available precontoured locking distal radius bridge plate can be used (**Fig. 3**). The authors' preference is the latter, as they are lower in profile, easier to place, and allow for the use of smaller screws. Metacarpal fixation with

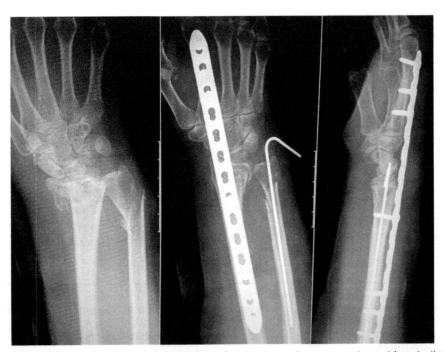

Fig. 1. A high-energy comminuted distal radius and ulna fracture in a polytrauma patient with an ipsilateral tibial plateau fracture and contralateral patella fracture, with interval dorsal spanning bridge plate application using a locking DCP, allowing immediate weight-bearing of the injured upper extremity on crutches.

A   **B**

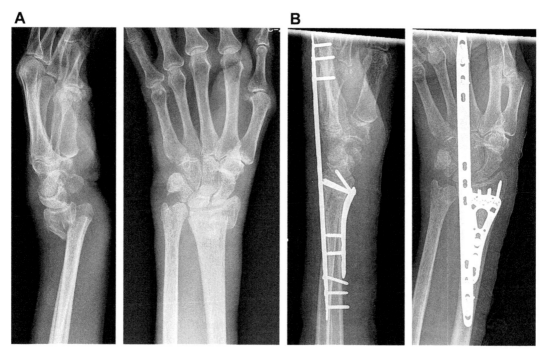

Fig. 2. (*A1, A2*) A low-energy fragility fracture of the distal radius in a walker-dependent patient who lives alone. (*B1, B2*) A dorsal spanning bridge plate was applied using a low-profile 2.7-mm locking dorsal spanning bridge plate, allowing immediate weight bearing with the injured upper extremity on the walker.

3.5-mm screws may be too large, and a screw diameter of 2.7 mm or smaller is preferable.

Patients are positioned supine with the injured arm extended onto a hand table. Either general and/or regional anesthesia can be used. The authors routinely use a tourniquet, but its application is optional. Intraoperative fluoroscopy is necessary. The fracture should be manipulated, and acceptable closed reduction of the distal radius

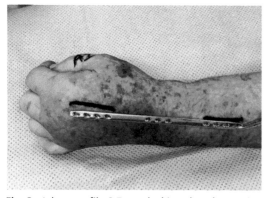

Fig. 3. A low-profile 2.7-mm locking dorsal spanning bridge plate (Depuy Synthes, West Chester, PA) applied to the dorsum of the injured wrist with the incisions marked for exposure and screw placement.

is confirmed with fluoroscopy. If necessary, Kirschner wires (K wires) or a freer can be introduced percutaneously to help aid in fracture reduction, with the ultimate goal being to maintain the fracture reduction with ligamentotaxis once internally fixed. Two incisions are marked out with the plate applied to the dorsal hand and wrist (see **Fig. 3**). Note that the distal incision is placed between the second and third metacarpals allowing for the option to apply the plate to either index or middle metacarpal. The authors' preference is to apply the plate to the index metacarpal, thereby fixing the wrist in slight ulnar deviation to help facilitate weight bearing with an assistive device.

The first incision is placed for the metacarpal fixation. Blunt dissection is taken down to the selected metacarpal. The extensor tendons are mobilized and retracted (**Fig. 4**). The metacarpal is exposed; a freer is introduced to create a path under the second or third compartments, for either plate fixation on the index or middle metacarpals, respectively (**Fig. 5**). The bridge plate is then slid retrograde under the selected compartment (**Fig. 6**). Attention is paid to confirm that the plate is placed under and not over the extensor tendons. Fluoroscopy is then used to confirm the appropriate provisional placement of the bridge plate. Once satisfied, the second incision is placed proximally with blunt dissection down to the radial

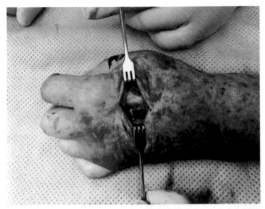

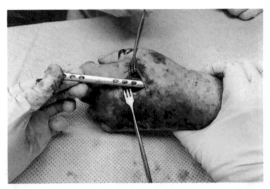

Fig. 6. The plate is inserted retrograde along the path created by the freer.

Fig. 4. With the extensor tendons retracted, the metacarpal is exposed.

shaft. If the plate is appropriately positioned, it will be found proximally between the extensor carpi radialis brevis and extensor pollicis longus tendons (**Fig. 7**).

The goal of internal fixation is 3 to 4 bicortical screws both proximally and distally, preferably with at least half being locking screws to increase the construct rigidity. Internal fixation begins with the placement of a nonlocking cortical screw distally in the metacarpal shaft first (**Fig. 8**). When the fracture is confirmed to be reduced with ligamentotaxis, a second nonlocking cortical screw is placed in the radial shaft proximally second (**Fig. 9**). Once satisfied with the fracture reduction and plate placement, the remaining screw holes are filled with locking screws (**Fig. 10**). Again, if the index metacarpal and the second compartment were selected for plate placement, the wrist will be fixed in slight ulnar deviation once the plate is internally fixed.

Following fixation, the skin incisions are closed in the standard fashion and a soft dressing is applied. Immediate weight bearing is allowed

and encouraged. Staged removal of the bridge plate is planned for 8 to 12 weeks later, once satisfied with the fracture union.

CASE SERIES

The authors had a series of 11 patients with a minimum follow-up of 1 year (range 12–27 months) treated with a dorsal spanning bridge plate who were all functional quadrupeds requiring immediate weight bearing with an assistive device. All cases were low-energy injuries consisting of falling from standing. The authors' average patient age was 72 years old (range 64–87 years). Fractures classified using the AO system yielded 1 A2, 3 A3, 2 C1, 2 C2, and 3 C3 patterns. All surgeries were performed under general anesthesia without infection or reoperation, except for the planned staged removal of hardware. However, before the planned removal of the hardware, there were 2 cases of implant fracture at the middle plate holes corresponding to the wrist joint, which were assumed to be from fatigue failure (**Fig. 11**). These cases were taken back for removal of the

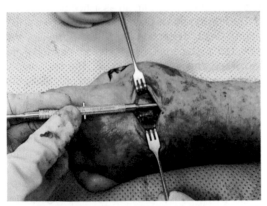

Fig. 5. A freer elevator is used to create a path under the extensor compartment in a retrograde fashion.

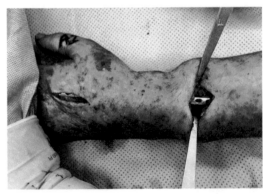

Fig. 7. Proximal exposure of the plate on the radial shaft should be directed between the interval of the extensor carpi radialis brevis and the extensor pollicis longus tendons.

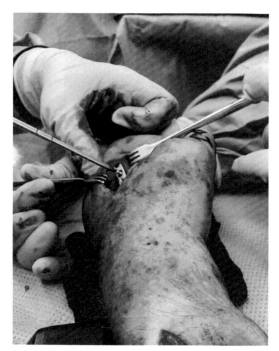

Fig. 8. Fixation begins distally with placement of a nonlocking cortical screw in the metacarpal shaft.

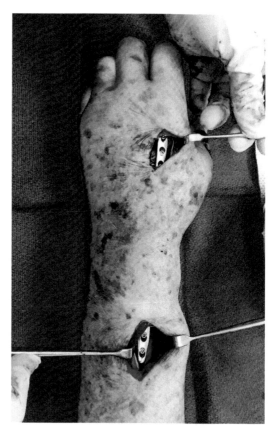

Fig. 10. Once satisfied with fracture reduction and plate fixation with a preliminary nonlocking cortical screw proximally and distally, the remaining plate holes are filled with locking screws to increase construct strength.

hardware earlier than planned, at approximately 8 weeks after their index surgery. For the remaining 9 cases, planned staged removal of the hardware was performed at 11 weeks on average (range 10–12). There were no cases of nonunion, tendon rupture, nerve injury or neuropraxia, or additional returns to the operating room beyond the planned staged of hardware removal.

DISCUSSION

In the authors' experience, treating patients with a distal radius fracture who are now functional quadrupeds with dorsal spanning plate fixation is a viable treatment option to improve or restore mobility with assistive devices. Intraoperatively, the treatment is straightforward, with the application of the plate requiring 2 small incisions and limited dissection, thereby limiting operative morbidity. Postoperatively, immediate weight bearing with the injured limb is allowed. Based on the authors' series, they now use low-profile

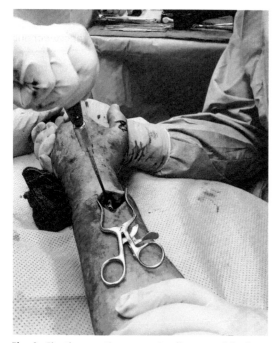

Fig. 9. Fixation continues proximally next with placement of a second nonlocking cortical screw in the radial shaft. Note the assistant applying gentle traction across the wrist to further reduce the distal radius fracture with ligamentotaxis.

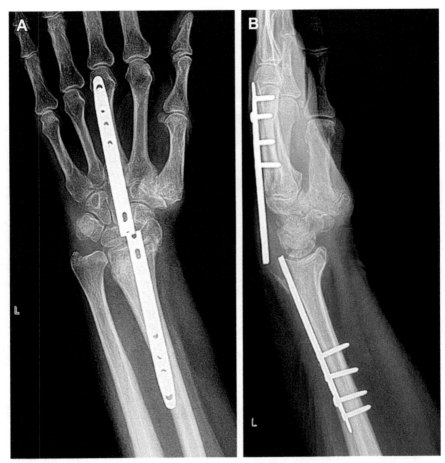

Fig. 11. Fatigue failure of the plate through the middle screw holes of the plate on the (A) anteroposterior and (B) lateral radiographs.

precontoured locking plates without midplate holes to avoid future fatigue fractures (**Fig. 12**).

In a prospective study by Ruch and colleagues,[9] 22 patients with comminuted distal radius fractures were treated with a dorsal spanning bridge plate and followed for at least 1 year, with an average age of 54 years (range 24–93 years). They included patients with high-energy distal

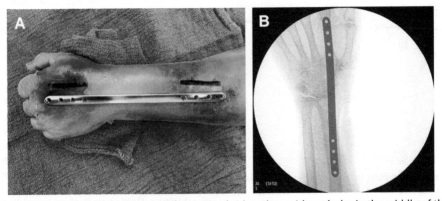

Fig. 12. (A) A low-profile 2.5-mm locking dorsal spanning bridge plate without holes in the middle of the plate to avoid fatigue failure of the plate with repetitive loading with weight bearing. (B) In situ, the lack of holes in the central portion are illustrated on fluoroscopy.

radius fractures with at least 4 cm of proximal diaphyseal extension. Patients were seen immediately postoperatively as well as at 6 months and 1 year postoperatively, with 18 patients also available at 2 years postoperatively. Nine of these patients had open fractures, with 2 requiring flap coverage. Postoperatively, patients were allowed to perform activities of daily living and had a 5-lb lifting restriction. Patients who had lower extremity injuries were allowed platform weight bearing only. In this series, all fractures healed with a mean time to hardware removal of 124 days. They reported no tendon ruptures and no cases of hardware failure. Although they had 3 infections, all were in patients with open fractures. They found no patients with digital stiffness; however, 3 patients had a 15 extensor lag while the plate was in place, which resolved after plate removal. When comparing this with the authors' patient cohort, it should be noted that these patients all had high-energy trauma, whereas in the authors' series, all patients had low-energy trauma with immediate full weight bearing allowed with the bridged upper extremity.

Richard and colleagues[11] performed a retrospective review of 33 patients older than 60 years with comminuted distal radius fractures treated with distraction plating. This study used a dorsal approach with a 2.5-mm or 3.5-mm DCP spanning plate. In 7 of these patients, supplemental K-wire fixation was also used. Patients were splinted postoperatively until suture removal and were given a 2-kg lifting restriction while the plate was in place. Patients were allowed to bear weight through the forearm if an assistive device was needed. The plates were removed at a mean of 119 days. All fractures healed, and there were no cases of tendon rupture. Ten patients developed digital stiffness, with one requiring tenolysis at the time of plate removal. In addition, there was one infection in a patient who had an open fracture during the initial injury. Patients were able to obtain a functional range of motion of the wrist with a mean flexion of 46° and mean extension of 50°; however, this was not compared with a control group or to the contralateral wrist.

Despite the advantage of immediate weight-bearing ability and consistent fracture healing using a dorsal spanning bridge plate for distal radius fractures, there are some disadvantages to this treatment algorithm. First, patients with a traditionally nonoperative fracture pattern would be undergoing a surgical procedure and are subject to the risks associated with surgery for plate placement and a second surgery for plate removal.

Second, as with any hardware, the plate and screws are subject to hardware failure or soft tissue irritation. In the authors' experience, they have also experienced plate fracture due to fatigue failure from repetitive loading and weight bearing. Fortunately, a plate fracture typically occurred 8 weeks after the index surgery when the fracture was already healed, thereby not altering postoperative weight-bearing allowance. However, based on this experience, the authors now preferentially use a 2.5-mm low-profile precontoured dorsal spanning bridge plate that does not have holes in the midsection of the plate to avoid fatigue fracture of the plate (see **Fig. 12**).

Third, stiffness of the wrist and fingers are of concern with prolonged immobilization of the wrist in neutral. In the authors' series, all patients underwent a gentle manipulation under anesthesia at their staged second surgery for removal of the plate and no patients required additional surgeries, including no interventions for loss of wrist motion. A previous meta-analysis and a later a prospective randomized trial comparing spanning external fixation with plate fixation confirm the authors' finding and also demonstrated no significant difference in wrist range of motion at 1 year.[12,13]

SUMMARY

Functional quadrupeds are patients who rely on their hands for weight bearing with an assistive device, such as walker-dependent patients and polytrauma patients. Dorsal spanning bridge plate fixation of distal radius fractures in functional quadrupeds is an effective surgical treatment option to facilitate immediate weight bearing through the injured wrist. This treatment benefits patients by allowing them earlier mobility and independence with their assistive devices. In the authors' series, patients have had satisfactory results. Further study is needed to assess the functional end points and patient satisfaction comparatively after dorsal spanning bridge plate fixation relative to other nonspanning fixation options as well as nonoperatively treated distal radius fractures in this patient population.

REFERENCES

1. Nellans KW, Kowalski E, Chung KC. The epidemiology of distal radius fractures. Hand Clin 2012; 28(2):113–25.
2. Baron JA, Karagas M, Barrett J, et al. Basic epidemiology of fractures of the upper and lower limb among Americans over 65 years of age. Epidemiology 1996;7(6):612–8.
3. Chung KC, Shauver MJ, Yin H, et al. Variations in the use of internal fixation for distal radial fracture in the United States Medicare population. J Bone Joint Surg Am 2011;93:2154–62.

4. Egol KA, Walsh M, Romo-Cardoso S, et al. Distal radial fractures in the elderly: operative compared with nonoperative treatment. J Bone Joint Surg Am 2010;92:1851–7.

5. Arora R, Lutz M, Deml C, et al. A prospective randomized trial comparing nonoperative treatment with volar locking plate fixation for displaced distal radial fractures in patients sixty-five years of age and older. J Bone Joint Surg Am 2011;93:2146–53.

6. Ilyas AM, Jupiter JB. Distal radius fractures–classification of treatment and indications for surgery. Hand Clin 2010;26(1):37–42.

7. Burke EF, Singer RM. Treatment of comminuted distal radius with the use of an internal distraction plate. Tech Hand Up Extrem Surg 1998;2: 248–52.

8. Dodds SD, Save AV, Yacob A. Dorsal spanning bridge plate fixation for distal radius fractures. Tech Hand Up Extrem Surg 2013;17:192–8.

9. Ruch DS, Ginn TA, Yang CC, et al. Use of a distraction plate for distal radial fractures with metaphyseal and diaphyseal comminution. J Bone Joint Surg Am 2005;87(5):945–54.

10. Hanel DP, Lu TS, Weil WM. Bridge plating of distal radius fractures: the Harborview method. Clin Orthop Relat Res 2006;445:91–9.

11. Richard MJ, Katolik LI, Hanel DP, et al. Distraction plating for the treatment of highly comminuted distal radius fractures in elderly patients. J Hand Surg Am 2012;37A:948–56.

12. Margaliot Z, Haase SC, Kotsis SV, et al. A meta-analysis of outcomes of external fixation versus plate osteosynthesis for unstable distal radius fractures. J Hand Surg Am 2005;30A:1185e1-17.

13. Egol K, Walsh M, Tejwani N, et al. Bridging external fixation and supplementary Kirschner-wire fixation versus volar locked plating for unstable fractures of the distal radius. J Bone Joint Surg Br 2008; 90-B:1214–21.

Moving?

Make sure your subscription moves with you!

To notify us of your new address, find your **Clinics Account Number** (located on your mailing label above your name), and contact customer service at:

Email: journalscustomerservice-usa@elsevier.com

800-654-2452 (subscribers in the U.S. & Canada)
314-447-8871 (subscribers outside of the U.S. & Canada)

Fax number: 314-447-8029

Elsevier Health Sciences Division
Subscription Customer Service
3251 Riverport Lane
Maryland Heights, MO 63043

ELSEVIER

Printed and bound by CPI Group (UK) Ltd, Croydon, CR0 4YY

03/10/2024

01040302-0007